Springer-Verlag Italia Srl.

Advances in Sports Cardiology

Edited by   A. Pelliccia
                      G. Caselli
                      P. Bellotti

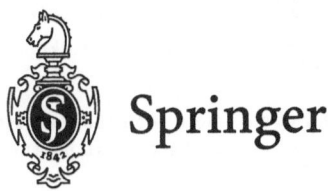 Springer

A. Pelliccia • G. Caselli • P. Bellotti
Comitato Olimpico Nazionale Italiano
Istituto di Scienza dello Sport
Scuola dello Sport
Via dei Campi Sportivi, 46
00197 Roma, Italy

ISBN 978-3-540-75036-9   ISBN 978-88-470-2298-0 (eBook)
DOI 10.1007/978-88-470-2298-0

Typesetting: Graphostudio, Milano

Contents

Foreword

The original articles included in the present book have primarily been taken from papers presented at the International Advanced Course, more precise the Master on Sports Cardiology, held in Rome from November 27 to December 15 1995 at the School of Sport and Institute of Sport Sciences of the Italian National Olympic Committee. The contributions, written by internationally acknowledged scientists, appeared after extensive and careful revision by the Authors, and represent current and highly profitable scientific material. The incentive to publish this work came from Springer-Verlag, a renowned publisher, and the articles have been compiled in Advances in Sports Cardiology.

The present volume is an easy-to-consult, comprehensive and up-to-date reference. Possible future developments in cardiovascular evaluation in athletes have been covered, too.

The cardiological evaluation of athletes represents a more than 30 years-old discipline in Italy, with legal implications, which compel physicians in this field to investigate in each individual athlete the possible, innermost causes of cardiovascular abnormality and to express a circumstantial prognostic assessment. Cardiologists in this field should have an extensive background in physiology but should also be aware of the indications and limits of the instrumental diagnostic procedures used in clinical practice as well as of the distinction between normal physiological adaptation to exercise and training and a true pathological cardiac process. Hence, sound basis in physiology with a major interest in clinical practice distinguishes sports cardiology as a new and original discipline.

Sports cardiology is undoubtedly still young, still striving to establish its scientific and professional identity. It will most certainly do so in an environment in which preventive medicine is a significant issue affecting the vast population of athletes young and old who represent our society.

The Editors

The Impact of Sports Cardiology on Clinical Practice

A. Dagianti

Department of Cardiorespiratory Diseases, University "La Sapienza" Rome, Italian Society of Sports Cardiology, Rome, Italy

Sports cardiology and clinical cardiology are similar in that they both deal with cardiovascular physiology. The former mainly concerns adaptations of the heart to physical exercise and the latter often deals with the morpho-functional changes in anatomy and physiology with respect to disease conditions both at rest and during exercise. For this reason the clinical cardiologist cannot ignore the wealth of cardiovascular physiology knowledge derived also from sports cardiology.

The discipline of sports cardiology is of real importance, not only for its in depth investigation of cardiovascular physiology, but also for its intrinsic clinical issues and the cultural aspects related to the modern society where there is increasing tendency to engage in sports.

Undoubtedly, sports cardiology tooks advantage of the observations on human cardiovascular physiology made in laboratories in Paris, Vienna, Berlin and also Italy at the end of the XIX and beginning of the XX century: among the most outstanding Italian physiologists we recall Mosso from Turin, Margaria and Cerretelli from Milan, Cerquiglini and Luciani from Rome. These Physiology Schools greatly contributed to the study of adaptations of the cardiovascular system to muscular exercise which, in turn, represented the reference point for clinical cardiology, the subsequent study of which gave improvements in the knowledge of sports cardiology.

The close correlation between these disciplines is confirmed by the concern the sports cardiologist has in distinguishing between normal and pathological condition as well as with the adaptations of the cardiovascular system that are often influenced also by psychologic adjustments.

Clinical cardiology has greatly benefitted from studies on the athlete's heart that, particularly in recent years and thanks, to investigations carried out within our School, have modified the clinical approach to cardiomegaly and myocardial hypertrophy. Early observations on the athlete's heart date from the XIX century, though from the beginning discussion was aroused as to whether changes were the result of a physiological adaptation of the heart to exercise or of a heart impairment following intense and prolonged physical activity.

A further advance in sports cardiology has been attained by using more sophisticated techniques. As stated by Rost cardiac ultrasound represented a fundamental step forward in cardiovascular knowledge, in addition to being extremely suitable for sports medicine. For the first time, in fact, echocardiography has allowed the non-invasive study of both cardiac morphology and function leading to an adequate evaluation of the modifications which occurr in the athlete's heart. The need for a combined morphological and functional analysis of cardiovascular adaptation to exercise arises from physiology itself: it is sufficient to recall Laplace's law that encompasses morphological and functional parameters, i.e. intraventricular blood pressure, ventricular volume and wall thickness.

This new study approach has recently allowed the identification of the true anatomo-functional behaviour of the athlete's heart. 20 years ago Morganroth, using M-mode echocardiography, distinguished two kinds of athlete's hearts, namely that of the endurance and that of the highly trained athlete. In contrast, using two-dimensional echocardiography, we have demonstrated that the adaptive response is mostly the same in all types of sport, due to the same training the athletes perform. However, when muscular activity calls for pressure increase, as in the case of resistance athletes, morphological adaptation results in ventricular longitudinal diameter stretching and unmodified or even reduced trasversal diameter by parallel duplicating sarcomeres; mass increase however always corresponds to volume increase. In endurance athletes, due to the huge venous reflow, fibers stretch by serial duplicating sarcomeres in accordance with the Maestrini-Starling law, there is an increase in volume, longitudinal and transversal diameters and myocardial mass. Surprisingly, these cardiovascular adaptations exist in nature; the giraffe's heart symbolizing the heart of resistance athletes and the amphibians heart comparable to that of endurance athletes, being representative of pressure overload and volume overload respectively.

Briefly, we can say that in the athlete's heart there occurs 1) a proportional volume and mass increase with a constant mass/volume ratio, and 2) a compliance increase demonstrated by original studies performed in our School on systo-diastolic modifications of the left ventricular diameter and velocity. Our findings have lead us to label the athlete's diastole as "supernormal" for its incredible functional adaptation with complete ventricular filling from proto-mesodiastole and poor filling during atrial systole necessary for high venous reflow during physical activity [1, 2].

All these advances in the knowledge of the athlete's heart have been of considerable diagnostic value to the clinician cardiologist, making it possible to demonstrate that cardiac adaptation where the mass/volume ratio remains constant does not occur in pathologic myocardial hypertrophy. In this condition, an increase in ventricular afterload leads to the mass/volume ratio exceeding unit. Besides the above-mentioned morpho-functional changes, it has been possible to show a reduction in wall stress and bradycardia which allows lower maximal oxygen consumption and higher cardiovascular performance. Conversely, pathologic conditions bring about increased wall stress and tachycardia leading to higher maximal oxygen consumption that is not always counterbalanced by an increase in oxygen supply from an enhanced coronary blood flow.

In this respect, it has been demonstrated that the highest cardiac performance is allowed by an improved oxygen supply to the myocardium, partially due to increased extraction, near maximum at rest, but mostly due to an enhanced coronary blood flow. Zeppilli observed by echocardiography, that coronary arteries increased in caliber in trained subjects, a finding which later confirmed by coronarographic studies [3]. Morphological observations match those findings, showing a functional improvement in the coronary circulation as a consequence of enhanced vasodilation and a better distribution of blood flow. Moreover, humoral and neuromodulators of the coronary circulation have been shown to modify coronary vascularization according to muscular activity. In the study of Haskell [4], for example, nitroderivatives with endothelium-dependent activity have been proven to have twice the efficacy on coronary circulation in trained subjects. This is in contrast with our findings in pathological conditions as, for example, in myocardial hypertrophy due to hypertension, in which morphological alterations of the coronary vessels occur characterized by tortuosity of the first and second range vessels. Tortuosity takes place in the presence of a high mass/volume ratio that is always absent in athletes. As per Poiseuille's law, increase in length and reduction in vessel caliber and tortuous vessel angle involve an increased resistance to blood flow at the level of the conductance vessels [5]. The modified morphology involved in the genesis of myocardial ischemia following hypertension seems to be due, on one hand, to the higher resistance to blood flow caused by the mass increase, and on the other to the functional disorder of intramyocardial vessels.

Thus the above-mentioned observations have led us to clearly distinguish between physiological myocardial hypertrophy from any other pathologic hypertrophic forms, and to consider muscular activity as a possible therapeutic means in hypertension and ischemic cardiopathy. In addition, they have provided new insights into cardiovascular physiology and improved clinical diagnosis. Thanks to the knowledge attained in the field of physiological remodelling, as occurring in the athlete's heart, we can update the definition of postinfarction ventricular remodelling as "new morpho-functional adaptation in response to the overturned topographic condition and altered ventricular geometry". Ventricular remodelling is therefore conceived as an anatomo-functional change capable of reaching higher functional performance with lower oxygen consumption.

A further fundamental step in the knowledge of the physiology of physical exercise and sports cardiology and the influence of the latter on clinical cardiology was the demonstration of the close relationship between VO_2, maximum heart rate and age. It is from this relationship that the concept of maximum VO_2 originated as the expression of maximum cardiovascular activity which, as the vector of O_2, represents the true factor limiting maximum physical performance. The wonderful adaptation of the "human machine" in modifying and improving itself can be expressed by the maximum aerobic power linked, in its turn, to cardiac reserve, expressed by the formula $VO_2 = Q \times (D\,A\text{-}VO_2) = Qs \times FC \times (D\,A\text{-}VO_2)$. It is sufficient to remember how, through this knowledge, it has been possible to differentiate maximal from sub-maximal performance and to recognize how these, to which the release of the cardiovascular activity from the neurovegetative system corresponds, can be used for diagnostic purposes. This is because they are examples of the modifications of the ventricular repolarization phase during muscular stress.

Another important aspect of sports cardiology, which made an important contribution to clinical cardiology, was the suitability of the cardiovascular system to sports activity and therefore the identification of cardiac pathologies at risk in the sports population This represents a crucial problem which closely unites clinical and sports cardiology. Furthermore, in some pathological states such as, for example, arrhythmogenic right ventricular dysplasia, Wolff-Parkinson-White syndrome, etc. that particularly affect young people frequently without symptoms and apparent cardiovascular normality, a great contribution, especially in the field of prognosis, came from the results of the necessary, widespread investigations in sports medicine, with important gains in clinical cardiology. Therefore, we can understand how collaboration between sports and clinical cardiology is of fundamental importance, especially for a modern, multiparametric, systematic approach. I believe that this is necessary and, moreover, now possible due to sophisticated investigation techniques, which must, however, be adapted to clinical application; otherwise there is a risk, frequently occurring with young physicians, of creating false "instrumental" illnesses. The sudden death of athletes on the field has often reproposed this topic. I believe that it fully concerns both sports and clinical cardiology, representing a crucial problem for both disciplines and a further demonstration of the close relationship between them.

The increased diffusion of sports activities among the population, with a particular increase in the older age group, has further broadened the clinical and physiological themes of sports cardiology until it encompasses the assessment of the effects and the eventual indication of physical activity in subjects with evident cardiovascular pathology. Even the physiologists who investigated the effects of sports activities in healthy subjects, with their well-documented observations, urged clinicians to use this sports-therapy. As previously noted, physical activity is capable of increasing coronary flow by anatomic and functional modifications. Rehabilitation in coronary artery disease has become of increasing importance because of the positive effects of physical exercise not only on myocardial oxygen supply and consumption, but also due to the improved use of O_2 in the periphery and the favourable changes induced in the autonomic nervous system. It should also be recalled how recent experiments performed in our school demonstrated that patients who had undergone coronary artery by-pass surgery and who were performing regular physical activity, 2-3 years after the surgical intervention had improved cardiac performance with higher cardiac output and showed a greater increase in coronary blood flow [6]. This is to be compared with patients who had undergone surgery but had a sedentary life style. It should be mentioned that in this last matter all now agree that the American Heart Association has recognized sedentary life style as a risk factor for independent and changeable heart disease and sports-therapy as a primary means of prevention. Thus increased activity, be it sports or recreational, is recognized as having the power to reduce the risk of cardiac death, especially from heart disease, in subjects without clinical symptoms indicating cardiopathy.

It therefore appears obvious that physical activity can improve cardiovascular performance and recently there is a tendency to believe that when carried out in later years it can keep people active for longer and possibly even lengthen lifes. Hence is born the more modern view, which needs to be duly developed in future studies, of the possibilities offered by physical activity in preventing the "illness" progression referred to as senescence. However the intimate mechanisms of action and the most appropriate time and means of application of what can be considered a therapeutic intervention, in the same way as pharmacological intervention, have yet to be clarified.

I hope that with what has been said it is evident that sports cardiology has assumed a scientific and cultural physionomy of its own fully involving expertise and sound knowledge, not only physiological, but also clinical cardiology.

References

1. Dagianti A, Penco M, Fedele F, Sciomer S, Fabietti F, Agati L, Pelliccia A, Zeppilli P (1988) Non invasive morphological and functional evaluation of athletes in Sports Cardiology. Int J Sports Cardiol 5:1
2. Agati L, Fedele F, Gagliardi MG, Sciomer S, Penco M (1985) A supernormal behaviour of echocardiographic diastolic data in athletes despite left ventricular hypertrophy. Int J Sports Cardiol 2:10
3. Zeppilli P, Rubino P, Manno V, Cameli S, Palmieri V, Gorra A (1987) Visualizzazione ecocardiografica delle arterie coronarie in atleti di resistenza. G Ital Cardiol 17:957
4. Haskell WL, Sims C, Myll J, Bortz WM, Goar FG, Alderman EL (1993) Coronary artery size and dilating capacity in ultradistance runners. Circulation 87:1076
5. Dagianti A, Rosanio S, Luongo R, Dagianti A jr, Fedele F (1993) Morfometria coronarica nell'ipertensione arteriosa essenziale. Cardiologia 38:497
6. Penco M, Fabietti F, Fedele F, Dagianti A (1989) Ruolo dell'esercizio fisico nel trattamento dei soggetti sottoposti a by-pass aorto-coronarico. "Heart Surgery 1989", CESI Ed., Roma, p.613

Cardiovascular Response and Adaptation to Exercise

J. H. Mitchell

Harry S. Moss Heart Center, University of Texas Southwestern Medical Center, Dallas, Texas, USA

Exercise can be classified into two broad categories according to mechanical activity and these are dynamic or isotonic and static or isometric. In dynamic exercise there are changes in muscle length and movements in joints caused by rhythmic muscle contractions which develop little tension. In static exercise there is a relatively large generation of muscle tension caused by contractions with little or no change in muscle length and little or no movement in joints. Physical activities such as long distance running or cross-country skiing (classic technique) are pure dynamic exercise and weight-lifting or water-skiing are pure static exercise. However, these two types of activity should be thought of as the two opposite poles of a continuum in which most physical activity has components of both static and dynamic exercise. For example, rowing and speed skating involve both dynamic and static exercise.

The classification of exercise by its mechanical action is different from characterizing the activity based on the type of metabolism that is utilized for the production of energy. In this way exercise can be categorized as aerobic when the energy comes from an oxidative process and anaerobic when the energy comes from a glycolytic process. In general, high intensity static exercise is performed primarily anaerobically and high intensity dynamic exercise lasting longer than several minutes is performed primarily aerobically. However, high intensity dynamic exercise for a brief period of time such as sprinting or jumping is performed primarily anaerobically.

Dynamic Exercise

Dynamic exercise involving a large muscle mass causes a large increase in oxygen consumption (Fig. 1). Cardiac output, heart rate, stroke volume and systolic arterial pressure increase markedly with only a small increase in mean arterial pressure. In addition, there is a moderate decrease in diastolic arterial pressure and a marked decrease in total peripheral vascular resistance. There is also a marked increase of the total body arteriovenous oxygen difference.

The most important measure of the ability to perform dynamic exercise is the maximal oxygen uptake (VO_2 max) which is the maximal rate of removal of oxygen from inspired air and its utilization by the contracting muscles. VO_2 max is the product of maximal cardiac output and maximal total body arterio-

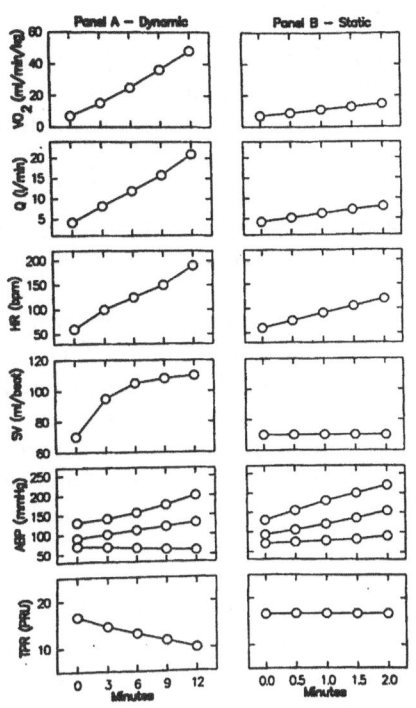

Fig. 1. Cardiovascular response to Exercise. Panel A. Effects of progressively increasing workload to VO$_2$max. Panel B. Effects of sustained isometric handgrip contraction (30% maximal voluntary contraction). VO$_2$ = oxygen consumption, Q = cardiac output, HR = heart rate, SV = stroke volume, APB = systolic (top line), mean (middle line) and diastolic (bottom line) arterial blood pressure, TPR = total peripheral resistance (from [9], Fig. 17.2)

venous oxygen difference (Fig. 2).

Maximal cardiac output is the product of the maximal heart rate and maximal stroke volume, and maximal total body arteriovenous oxygen difference is the arterial oxygen content minus the mixed venous oxygen content. During

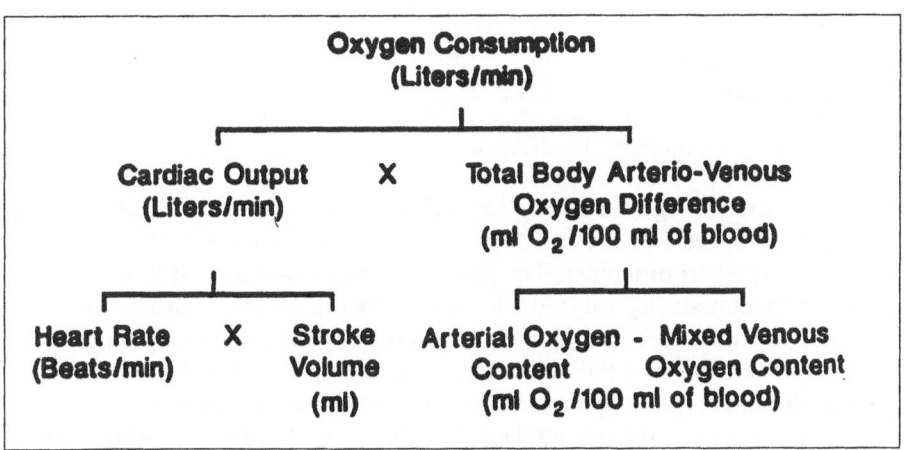

Fig. 2. Determinants of maximal oxygen consumption (VO$_2$max)

maximal exercise the mixed venous oxygen content can decrease to 3 to 4 $mlO_2/100$ ml blood. The extent to which the mixed venous O_2 content can fall is dependent upon the redistribution of blood flow away from inactive tissue and the degree of extraction of oxygen from the blood perfusing contracting muscles.

Maximal oxygen uptake (VO_2max) sets the limit of endurance performance for an individual. However, the ability to utilize a high percentage of VO_2max for a prolonged period of time is also of great importance. Thus endurance performance is not dependent only on $V0_2$max.

Training utilizing dynamic exercise or endurance training elicits cardio-vascular adaptation which are present both at rest and during exercise (Table I). Resting cardiac output is not changed by endurance training, but heart rate is decreased (training bradycardia) with a concomitant increase in stroke volume. Endurance training may cause a decrease in resting blood pressure. At the same submaximal workload, which after endurance training is a lower relative work-load, the cardiac output is the same but is achieved by having a lower submaxi-mal heart rate and a larger submaximal stroke volume.

Table 1. Effects of endurance training on oxygen consumption and hemodynamics

	Rest	Same Submaximal Workload	Maximal Workload
Oxygen consumption	↔	↔	↑
Cardiac output	↔	↔	↑
AVO₂ difference	↔	↔	↑
Heart rate	↓	↓	↔
Stroke volume	↑	– ↑	↑
Left ventricular Contractility	↔	↔	↑
Muscle blood flow	↔	↔	↑
Splanchnic blood flow	↔	↔	↓
Oxygen extraction	↔	↔	↑

↔ = no change, ↑ = increase, ↓ = decrease

The maximal oxygen consumption and maximal workload are higher after endurance training. This is due to a greater maximal cardiac output and a grea-ter total body AVO_2 difference. The greater maximal cardiac output is due to a greater maximal stroke volume with no change in maximal heart rate. The greater AVO_2 difference during maximal exercise is due to a greater blood flow and oxygen extraction in the working muscles and to a greater decrease in flow to the abdominal organs (splanchnic blood flow) and to the kidneys.

The magnitude of the maximal stroke volume is related to the degree of left ventricular eccentric hypertrophy that has been achieved. Left ventricular mass is greater in male and female endurance trained athletes than in sedentary control subjects (Fig. 3). This is also true when left ventricular mass is normalized to lean body mass.

The degree of left ventricular eccentric hypertrophy is due both to a genetic factor and to the duration and intensity of the endurance training. It has also been shown that the magnitude of left ventricular eccentric hypertrophy correlates with maximal oxygen consumption (Fig. 4).

In addition to increasing the maximal oxygen consumption, endurance training also enhances the ability to maintain a high percentage of VO_2 for a longer period of time. Both of these are important for enhanced endurance performance.

Static Exercise

Static exercise causes only a small increase in oxygen consumption during the activity even when a large muscle mass in involved (Fig. 1). After cessation of the activity there is a greater increase in oxygen consumption. There is a small increase in cardiac output and heart rate with no change in stroke volume. In addition, there is a marked increase in systolic, diastolic and mean arterial pressure with no appreciable change in total peripheral resistance. The magnitude of the increase in blood pressure is related to the intensity of the muscle contraction (% of maximal voluntary contraction) and to the amount of skeletal muscle involved in the exercise. There is also a small increase in the total body arteriovenous oxygen difference during the exercise and a greater increase immediately upon completion of the activity.

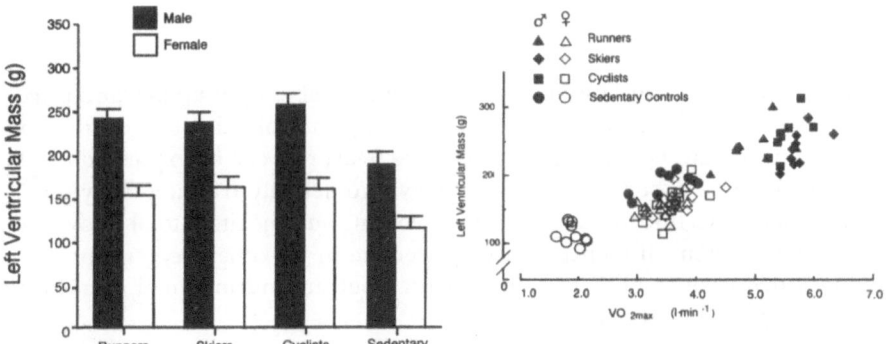

Fig. 3. Left ventricular mass of male and female sedentary controls and endurance trained athletes (from [9], Fig. 17.10)

Fig. 4. Relation of left ventricular mass in grams (g) to maximal oxygen uptake (VO_2max) in male and female sedentary controls and endurance trained athletes (from [9], Fig. 17.11)

Training utilizing static exercise or strength training causes an increased skeletal muscle mass due primarily to fiber hypertrophy with a small contribution from fiber hyperplasia (by 15%). This type of training, however, does not result in a higher maximal oxygen uptake. With pure strength training there appears to be some degree of left ventricular concentric hypertrophy. This type of adaptation allows a lesser wall force for the high left ventricular pressures that are present during static exercise. When left ventricular mass is indexed by lean body mass there is no difference between strength athletes and normal subjects.

Effects of Gender

In general, the cardiovascular response to dynamic and static exercise is qualitatively similar in men and women. However, there does appear to be a difference in the quantitative response of the cardiovascular system. It has been shown that men have larger blood volumes and increased oxygen carrying capacity of blood. In addition, studies using magnetic resonance imaging have shown that both sedentary and endurance trained men have larger left ventricular masses than do sedentary and endurance trained women. This is true both in absolute terms (Fig. 3) and when indexed by body weight or lean body mass. Maximal heart rates are similar in men and women. However, men can reach higher maximal oxygen uptakes than women because of larger maximal stroke volumes and larger maximal total body arterio-venous oxygen differences.

The response to dynamic exercise training in a qualitative sense is relatively the same for men and women. However, there are quantitative differences in the response of blood volume, stroke volume and left ventricular eccentric hypertrophy.

Effects of Age

With age there is a progressive decrease in maximal oxygen uptake and a reduced performance in dynamic exercise. This is principally due to a decrease in maximal heart rate. On average, the maximal heart rate can be expressed as 220 age. This decline occurs in both sedentary and actively training individuals. There is also a decline in maximal stroke volume and maximal total body arterio-venous oxygen difference. Thus the decline in maximal oxygen uptake is due to a decrease in both maximal cardiac output and maximal total body arterio-venous oxygen difference.

Neural Control during Exercise

There are two neural mechanisms which play important roles in determining the cardiovascular response to exercise (Fig. 5). In one of these, the neural activity which is responsible for the recruitment of motor units in the cortex activates, in parallel, the cardiovascular control areas in the medulla. This feedforward mechanism which determines the immediate changes in the level of parasympathetic and sympathetic efferent neural activity to the heart and blood vessels has been termed central command.

In the other neural mechanism, stimulation of mechanoreceptors and chemically sensitive metaboreceptors in the contracting skeletal muscle reflexly activates the same cardiovascular control areas in the medulla. This feedback mechanism, which can also determine the autonomic efferent activity, has been termed the exercise pressor reflex.

Nerve impulses related to the mechanical activity within the skeletal muscle are transmitted primarily by the thinly myelinated Group III afferents

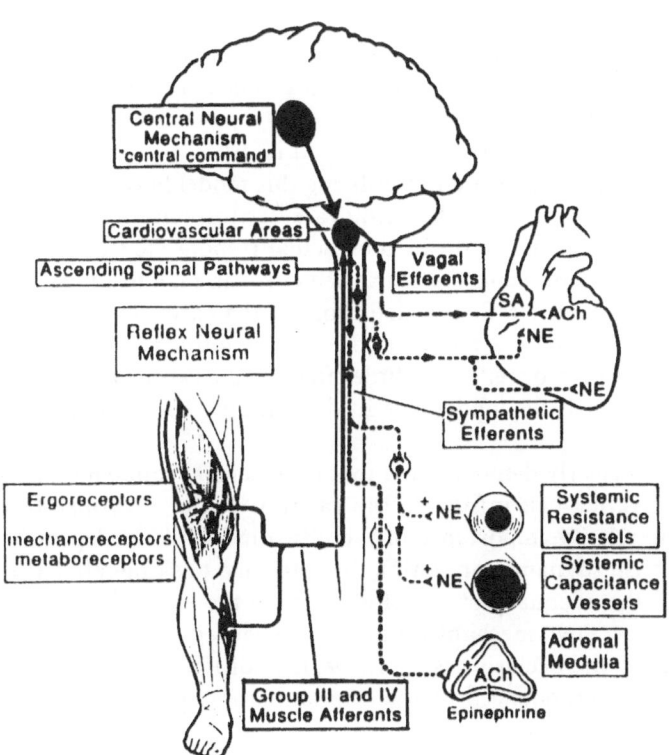

Fig. 5. Neural control of the circulation during exercise (From [10])

and neural impulses related to the metabolic activity within the skeletal muscle are transmitted primarily by the unmyelinated Group IV afferents. Both Group III and IV muscle afferents travel through the dorsal horn into the spinal cord and ascend to the cardiovascular control areas in the medulla.

The afferent nerve traffic from the activation of mechanoreceptors reaches the control areas in the medulla slightly later than neural impulse from central command. Central command can increase the heart rate within the first beat even when exercise is initiated in the last third of a cardiac cycle. The reflex from muscle mechanoreceptors can only increase the heart rate within the first beat when exercise is initiated in the first third of a cardiac cycle. With both of these mechanisms the initial increase in heart rate is due to parasympathetic withdrawal. Later the heart rate is also increased by sympathetic activation. Both central command and a reflex mechanism from mechanoreceptors provide information concerning the type and intensity of the muscle activation and the mass of skeletal muscle involved in the exercise. The afferent nerve traffic from the activation of metaboreceptors depends on an increase in concentration of some metabolite(s) that is (are) produced by the increased activity of the contracting muscle and, therefore, these neural signals are slightly delayed in reaching the cardiovascular control areas. Substances that have been proposed as the metabolic signal are potassium, hydrogen ion and adenosine.

In man neuromuscular blockade has been used to study the influence of central command in determining the cardiovascular response to both dynamic and static exercise.

This manoeuvre increases the perceived effort to perform a given level of dynamic or static exercise. Studies utilizing this model have shown that central command has little effect on the cardiovascular response to dynamic exercise but a more marked effect on the cardiovascular response to static exercise.

In addition, epidural anesthesia has been used in man to study the influence of the exercise pressor reflex in determining the cardiovascular response to both dynamic and static exercise. Studies utilizing this procedure have shown that the exercise pressor reflex has little effect on the cardiovascular response to static exercise but is of importance in determining the response to dynamic exercise.

It has been clearly demonstrated that both central command and the exercise pressor reflex can influence the cardiovascular response to exercise. However, the relative importance of these two mechanisms depends upon the type of exercise (dynamic or static), the intensity, the time after the onset of exercise and the adequacy of the blood flow to the exercising muscle. Also it appears that these two mechanisms are somewhat redundant, rather than additive, and that neural occlusion is operative. In addition, cardiovascular response during exercise is influenced by the arterial baroreceptors and the cardiopulmonary receptors.

Suggested Readings

1. Asmussen E (1981) Similarities and dissimilarities between static and dynamic exercise. I-3-I 17, Circulation Research 48 (Suppl I): I-3-17
2. Snell PG, and JH Mitchell (1984) The role of maximal oxygen uptake in exercise performance. Clinics in Chest Medicine 5:51-62
3. Mitchell JH, Tate C, Raven P, Cobb F, Kraus W Moreadith R, O'Toole M, Saltin B, and Wagner N (1992) Acute response and chronic adaptation to exercise in women. Medicine and Science in Sports and Exercise 24(6):S258-S265
4. Smith ML, and JH Mitchell (1993) Cardiorespiratory adaptations to exercise training. In: ACSM's Resource Manual for Guidelines for Exercise Testing and Prescription. 2nd Ed, SN Blair, P Painter, RR Pate, LK Smith, CB Taylor (Eds.) for the American College of Sports Medicine, Philadelphia, Lea & Febiger pp 75-81
5. Mitchell JH: The anatomy of the athlete's heart. In (1994) The Big Heart: Proceedings of a Course Held at the International School of Medical Sciences, AA Raineri and RD Leachman (Eds), Chur Switzerland, Harwood Academic Publishers pp 49-57
6. Mitchell JH (1994) The systolic and diastolic function of the athlete's heart. In The Big Heart: Proceedings of a Course Held at the International School of Medical Sciences AA, Raineri and RD Leachman (Eds), Chur, Switzerland, Harwood Academic Publishers pp 73-85
7. Mitchell JH, and PB Raven (1994) Cardiovascular adaptation to physical activity. In: Physical Activity, Fitness and Health: International Proceedings and Consensus Statement, C Bouchard, R Shephard, T Stephens (Eds), Champaign, Illinois, Human Kinetics Publishers pp 286-298
8. Mitchell JH, Haskell WL, Raven PB (1994) Classification of sports. Journal of the American College of Cardiology 24:864-866, October, 1994; Medicine and Science in Sports and Exercise, 26(10):S242-S245
9. Mitchell JH and Raven PB (1994) Cardiovascular response and adaptation to exercise. In: Physical Activity, Fitness and Health: International Consensus Statement, Bouchard C, Shephard R and Stephens T (Eds), Champaign, IL: Human Kinetics Publishers, pp 286-298
10. Mitchell JH (1990) Joseph B. Wolffe Memorial Lecture, Medicine and Science in Sports and Exercise, 22:141-154

Functional Evaluation in Sports Cardiology

M. Faina, A. Dal Monte, G. Mirri

Institute of Sport Sciences, Dept. of Physiology and Biomechanics,
C.O.N.I., Rome, Italy

In sports cardiology, the specific functional evaluation of athletes has assumed an increasingly important role in the development of in clinical and physiological analysis techniques and in the knowledge of adjustments and adaptations of the cardiovascular system when subjected to training loads.

Therefore, at present, while the aim is to make a "specific cardiological diagnosis" and at the same time detect the physiological parameters "useful for a specific functional evaluation", the sports cardiologist's primary objective of is to verify the behaviour of the cardiovascular system either directly during competitions, or in conditions as close as possible to competition in order to obtain responses that are undetectable with non-specific methodology.

Accordingly, in the case of laboratory evaluation, the basic assumption is to reproduce the biomechanical and physiological conditions of athletes during official competitions. The so-called specific ergometers have been for this purpose, used for some time. They are apparatus which give the possibility of simulating the specific technical action; therefore they allow the assessment of the organic and functional response of athletes in conditions similar to those found in the sport [1].

In the case of evaluations carried out directly on the field, the basic assumption is to have instruments that permit us to analyse physiological parameters during real or simulated competitions, specific training sessions or competition heats, without considerably interfering with the performance of athletes.

Enormous progress has been made in the area of functional evaluation, by introducing modern miniaturized telemetric metabolic charts for measuring oxygen uptake and field instruments that measure blood lactate [2, 3].

Furthermore, it seems clear that experiments in the laboratory or carried out on the field, must analyse many parameters among which those related to or limited by the cardiovascular system.

Therefore, in this chapter we describe the physiological parameters, to be analysed both by physiologists and cardiologists, fundamental in evaluating cardiovascular efficiency.

Maximum Oxygen Uptake

The maximum speed with which the body can develop energy through the oxidative system, or the maximum power of aerobic metabolism, is commonly defined as maximum oxygen uptake (VO_2max).

High levels of VO2max are typical of athletes practising endurance or middle-distance sports in a non-homogeneous subject group (sprinters to endurance athletes), the value of VO_2max is directly related to the performance capacity during an endurance competition [4, 5].

VO_2max is a parameter of basic importance, from a clinical point of view, since it is a complete and integrated measure of all the mechanisms from the transportation O_2 rigth up to its utilization inside mitochondria. If this integration of physiological mechanisms is altered by pathological factors or by sedentary life style, the VO_2max is also negatively influenced.

Among the central and peripheral factors limiting the VO_2max, those of fundamental importance are the central cardiovascular factors to be identified in cardiac output ($\dot{Q}$) and the capacity of blood to combine and transport O_2 to the peripheral system (Hb content).

In fact when large muscular masses are involved, these factors (Hb content multiplied by SV) can contribute up to 80% in determining the VO_2max value, while peripheral aspects (diffusion capacity of blood and mitochondria enzymes) only 20%. Both factors reach values of 50% when the dimensions of the muscular masses involved are modest [6].

Because Q is given by the product of heart rate (HR) and stroke volume (SV), heart rate gives a rapid and rough estimation of central adaptation to the training load, is still a particularly important index for evaluation. In fact, a HR reduction at constant metabolic power is considered as the expression of an increase in stroke volume. Furthermore, the evaluation of HR, together with the related oxygen uptake, allows calculation of the relationship between the two parameters and consequent extrapolation give the corresponding O_2 uptake from the HR measured on the field. In fact, it is well-known that the correlation between HR and O_2 uptake, considered linear, is equal for everyone when expressed in percentage with respect to maximum values, but is absolutely individual when expressed in absolute value.

The Anaerobic Threshold

Much lactate is produced at work loads corresponding to the VO_2max. This metabolite progressively accumulates in the muscular regions involved, and the consequent increase of H^+ content causes fatigue (acute) and makes it impossible to continue the effort.

Therefore, at an intensity equal to the maximum aerobic power, physical exercise can be carried out for only a short period of time. The maximum duration is defined as a time limit or maximal aerobic intensity or time of VO2max exhaustion, it varies between 4 and 11 minutes [7].

In contrast, the maximum work load that can be carried out by a person for a prolonged period of time corresponds to a work intensity which does not cause an accumulation of lactate, therefore an intensity which is necessarily lower than the VO_2max. This maximum work intensity, varying depending on the characteristics of the athlete and of his/her training state, was defined as the aerobic-anaerobic threshold by Wasserman in 1964 between 60 and 90% of VO_2max, and more simply as the anaerobic threshold (AT) by Mader in 1976. It is identified as the point in the lactate/intensity of the work load curve which, corresponds to a blood lactate value of 4 mM [8, 9].

So, the anaerobic threshold expresses the work intensity beyond which aerobic metabolism can meet the energy demand no longer alone. Above this the production of ATP is guaranteed also by the glicolitic anaerobic metabolism with the consequent progressive accumulation of lactate in the blood.

In defining the anaerobic threshold, the term accumulation instead of production of lactate is used. According to some authors it is preferable to use the term Maximal Lactate Steady State (MLSS). It seems that this term in fact, better describes, from a biological point of view, what really happens during work "carried out at threshold intensity" which is a situation of maximum balance between the muscular lactate production (rate of apparition = Ra) and its elimination (rate of disappearance = Rd) is reached [10].

. The empirical observation has shown that on average the MLSS also is detected at a value of 4 mM.

However, fixing a single value of lactate which corresponds to the MLSS for everybody, as normally happens for the anaerobic threshold, seems biologically wrong. In fact, it has been shown that lactate values corresponding to the MLSS, generally vary between individuals from 3 to 5.5 mM (they rarely exceed 7 mM).

In any case, the discriminating factor of this parameter is that, on one hand, less lactate is produced and, on the other, more lactate is broken down at muscular level. So, the main limit seems essentially determined by the improvement of   peripheral muscular capacities to acquire and use O_2 even if there is no actual agreement on which biological mechanisms determine the inbalance in the ratio between production and metabolism. On the other hand, the capacity of transporting oxygen (efficiency of the cardiac pump and of the haemoglobin system) and the capacity of removing lactate by the capillary system (efficiency of the peripheral microcirculation) are equally important in setting this value. So, it is evident that in a situation of exclusive aerobic work, such as that taking place at the anaerobic threshold, the role played by the efficiency of the cardiovascular system, including its central and peripheral components, certainly is not marginal. Consequently, detecting the anaerobic threshold is a fundamental element in evaluating the peripheral and central adaptation to the training load. Moreover, it should be remembered that the determination of this parameter generally does not involve a maximal test and consequently can be executed in old people or in conditions of non perfect health with relatively higher tranquility.

Now we will illustrate the test protocols and their interpretation for evaluating the described functional parameters.

Laboratory Tests for Evaluating VO₂max

In evaluating VO_2max, it is necessary to use instruments capable of real-time measurement of pulmonary ventilation and the percentage of O_2 in the ventilated air (F_EO_2). The product of these two elements, corrected by appropriate indices (i.e. F_ECO_2, Step), determines the measure of VO_2.

From a methodological point of view, certain fundamental criteria concerning performance specificity and the protocol used carrying out laboratory tests for detecting the VO_2max are to be respected (this is valid in general also for the other parameters) [1].

Concerning the first aspect, the athlete who undergo a test should not be fatigued, must not have drunk alcoholic drinks, taken drugs or food or smoked and must have appropriately warmed up. The temperature must not exceed 20 degrees and humidity must be such (50-60%) as to permit good evaporation.

Concerning specificity, as mentioned before it is fundamental to use specific ergometers [1].

Moreover, one should remember that even if the well-known step test is not a good instrument for the specific functional evaluation of all sports, it remains, due to its praticality, an ergometer valid in sports cardiology especially when due a great number of test are to be carried out and specific heart and circulatory pathologies are not being analysed.

Concerning the test protocol, generally in maximal tests a triangular protocol is used which consists of progressively increasing the work load to the subject exhaustion.

To assess VO_2max protocols using sufficiently long steps to obtain the steady state for that load should be used, but they must be, as for as possible, of short overall duration (8-10 smin) with fast (each step = 1 min) increases of the work load with high increases of load to avoid phenomena of local fatigue. In our Institute longer steps are used (2 min) in a temptative to assess also a steady rate of energy production at each step.

To define the moment to interrupt the test, some people assume that the VO_2 max is reached when the VO_2 does not increase despite further load increases (Plateau) or at high lactatemia levels (8 mM) or when R values are higher than 1.15 or, finally, when the prefixed theoretic HRmax percentages are reached.

However, all these criteria were defined with subjects and protocols no longer used in Functional Evaluation laboratories. For this reason, we and other Authors think it is preferable to carry on the test until the athlete is exhausted, considering the maximum VO_2 value reached as VO_2max, which should more correctly be defined as the VO_2 peak.

This kind of test, among other things, involves the athlete totally, in particular from the psychological point of view.

On the Field Tests for Evaluating the VO_2max

When no instrument for directly measuring the F_EO_2 is available, indirect tests, which can be of submaximal and maximal type, are used. These are based on the assumptions that: 1) all people have the same mechanical efficiency (25%) in cycling or energy cost of running 4 $KJ•(Km•m)^{-1}$, independently of speed, and 2) for submaximal test only there is a linear correlation between HR and the intensity of the muscular work expressed as VO_2 [13].

The simplest submaximal tests include two bouts using the cycle-ergometer or the treadmill where HR is measured, in the final phase (steady state).

The HR values detected under each submaximal load are correlated with the corresponding VO_2, which is indirectly calculated from the mechanical power; assuming, as said before, that efficiency or energy cost of the muscular work are equal in everyone (for this purpose adequately prepared conversion tables are used). Thanks to the two points obtained it is possible to draw a linear correlation between HR and VO_2, (which is subjective) and expresses the aerobic characteristics of an individual [13].

. The VO_2max is calculated by extrapolating the line up to the HRmax of the individual examined, this value's, not directly measured and could be assumed to be 220 minus age. As for all indirect methods, the one described has a possibility of error due to the many theoretical assumptions it requires.

One of the main evaluation errors in indirectly determining the above-described VO_2max occurs in assuming the theoretical HRmax. This can be avoided by measuring the real HRmax of the individual and also by administering a maximal load test which makes the subject reach the "real" HRmax. However, in the case of aged or cardiopatic subjects this may not be advisable.

In cases where it is possible to carry out maximal tests, other simple evaluation protocols have been conceived, in which the VO_2max can be estimated on the maximal value of mechanical power.

These protocols require the performance maximal tests by using cycle-ergometers or treadmills, characterized by progressive increase of work loads until the individual is exhausted. The important characteristic is that they are extremely adaptable and thus applicable to athletes, healthy non athletes and cardiopathic patients simply by adapting, depending an the circumstances, the entity and method of increasing work loads.

Even if the indirect tests described for determining the VO_2max provide data which has a certain implicit error, they are easily applicable methods, particularly useful when numerous individuals are to be checked and, in any way, when the expensive and sophisticated instruments necessary for directly measuring the VO_2 are not available [4, 5].

On the other hand, technological evolution with the introduction of miniaturized telemetric metabolic charts has simplified the direct measurement of VO_2 also on the field [2, 3].

The advantages of using these instruments (e.g. K4 Cosmed) mainly consist in analysing the behaviour of the integrated mechanisms determining the

VO2max directly while the athlete executes his/her training exercises or even during competitions without considerably interfering with the sports action. Even from a clinic cardiological point of view, especially concerning the evaluation of the adaptation processes in individuals being rehabilitated, these new instruments can offer interesting perspectives.

Laboratory Tests for the Anaerobic Threshold

Based a what was said earlies, for the concept of anaerobic threshold, one sees that in an increasing-load test the work intensity passes from a submaximal phase lower than the anaerobic threshold to a maximal phase which exceeds it. So, measuring the variations in the different physiological parameters caused by this transition can provide an index of the anaerobic threshold itself.

Obviously, the physiological parameter best correlated with the anaerobic threshold is lactacidemia. Moreover, this parameter began to be used to identify the anaerobic threshold only after 1976, with the spread of the micro-methods of analysis and following Mader's suggestion of considering the work-load corresponding to the experimentally determined value, of 4 mM of blood lactate as the anaerobic threshold intensity. Before then, the only method used was based on detecting the variation of ventilation compared to that of VO_2. In fact, ventilation has a linear relationship with VO_2, up to a certain work load, considered as corresponding to the Anaerobic threshold, beyond which ventilation increases more than VO_2 [8, 9].

Many other methods have been described in the literature to assess the anaerobic threshold. Therefore, more complete information is available [14, 15].

On Field Tests for the Anaerobic Threshold

Conconi has proposed a on field test linking the heart rate to running speed in which the HR or the speed of the anaerobic threshold are indicated, at the point where the linear relationship between these two parameters is lost [16].

Some believe that Conconi's test is highly correlated with the real anaerobic threshold while others say this correlation is low.

This test is favoured because it is easy and practical to perform, while its negative aspects are the subjectivity in detecting the inflection point of HR and the fact that this inflection point is not always verifiable. Even if some specific mathematical analysis is used, a number of subjects who do not show the downward inflation of HR persists [17]. It is also to be considered that, since the HR of the anaerobic threshold is often used for on-line training control, that this parameter is not stable in time. It is subjected to variations completely independent from the intensity of the work load administered and due to factors such as the increase of body temperature and the possible occurrence of dehydration.

The test proposed by Mader can also be carried out on field. It consists of incremental step test, whose step duration is 5-6 minutes. Blood sample is withdrawn in the recovery period (30s) between the steps, each of them is performed at costant speed.

It is, all things considered, a normal increasing-load test not carried out until exhaustion since it only aims to point out the passage of the blood lactate curve through the 4mM value. Considering the wide variety of transportable instruments for determining lactacidemia this test, can be considered a field one, is highly correlated with MLSS.

References

1. Dal Monte A, Lupo S (1989) Specific ergometry in functional assessment of top class sportsmen. J Sport Med Phys Fitness 29:1
2. Dal Monte A, Sardella F, Alippi B, Faina M, Manetta A (1994) A new respiratory valve system for measuring oxygen uptake during swimming. Eur J Appl Physiol 69:159
3. Faina M, Pistelli R, Franzoso G, Petrelli G, Dal Monte A (1996) Validity and reliability of a new telemetric portable system with CO2 Analyzer (K4 Cosmed). Proceedings of 1d Congress of European College of Sport Science, Nizza, 572 (Abstract)
4. McArdle WD, Katch FI, Katch VL (1986) Exercise Physiology. Lea & Febiger ed. Philadelphia
5. Astrand PO, Rodahl K (1986) Textbook of work physiology. McGraw Hill ed, New York
6. Di Prampero PE(1985) Metabolic and circulatory limitations to VO2max at the whole animal level. J Exp Biol 115:319
7. Billat V, Renaux JC, Pinoteau J, Petit B, Koralsztein JP (1994) Times to exhaustion at 100% of velocity at VO2 max and modelling of the time - limit/velocity relationship in elite long-distance runners. Eur J Appl Physiol 69:271-273
8. Wassemann K, McIlory MB (1964) Detecting the threshold of anaerobic metabolism in cardiac patients during exercise. Am J Cardiol 14:44
9. Mader A, et al (1976) Zur beurteilung der Sporttarspezifischen Ausdaureleis tungsfahigkeit im Labor. Sprtaz. Sportmed 1:13
10. Brooks GA (1985) Anaerobic threshold: review of the concept and direction for the future. Medicine and Science in Sport and exercise 17: 22
11. Shepard RJ(1984) Text of Maximum Oxygen Intake A critical review. Sport medicine 1:99
12. Taylor HL, Buskirk E, Henschel A (1955) Maximal oxygen intake as an objective measure of cardiorespiratory performance. J Appl Physiol 8:73-80
13. Lamb DR (1984) Physiology of exercise Mac Millan
14. Moritani T et al (1981) Critical power as a measure of physical work capacity and anaerobic threshold. Ergonomics 24 (5) 339
15. Billiat V, Dalmay F, Antonini MT, Ghassain AP (1994) A method for determining the maximal lactate steady state of blood lactate concentration from two levels of submaximum exercise. Eur. J Appl Physiol 69:196
16. Conconi F, Ferrari M, Ziglio PG, Draghetti P, Codeca L (1982) Determination of the anaerobic threshold by a non invasive field test in runners. J Appl Physiol 52:869-873

17.   Mahmet K, Hakki G, Cem B, Neyhan E, Kagan U, and Huseyn U (1996) Determination of the heart rate deflrction point by the Dmax method. J Sports Med Phys Fitness36:31-4

Cardiovascular Adjustments in Wheelchair Paraplegic Athletes (WPA)

M. Marchetti

Human Physiology, Post Graduate School of Sport Medicine, University "La Sapienza", Rome, Italy

Paraplegic and tetraplegic patients constitute a great part of wheelchair dependent athletes. Although the benefits of sport in these subjects have been reported by a large number of authors, this presentation will stress that the anatomical and functional peculiarities of a para- or tetraplegic person are so unlike those of an able bodied subject that only very specialised trainers or sports physicians, well aware of those differences, can effectively take care of these athletes.

Heavy exercise in able bodied athletes (AA) produces a massive readjustment of circulation as summarised in the following scheme.

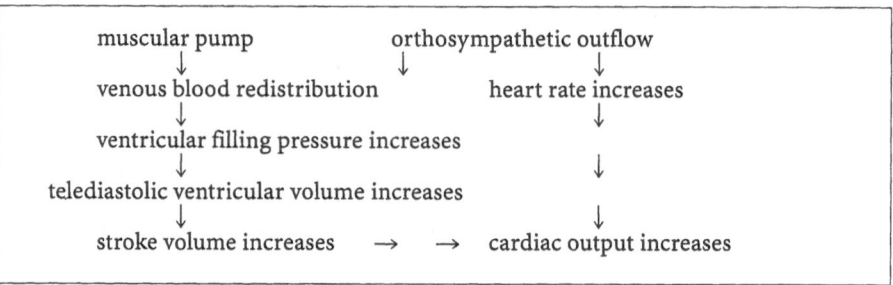

Fig. 1. AA cardiovascular adjustment to exercise

This adjustment, aimed at increasing blood flow in the active muscle and in thermo dissipating skin, implies a) a complex system of encephalic centers hierarchically organised which needs b) to receive a flow of information coming from every part of the body and c) to send commands to every part of the body. The interruption of the spinal cord denies this input/output flow from/to that part of the body associated with the spinal cord below the level of the lesion. This impairment is effective as high and/or complete as the interruption. The paraplegic condition can be summarised as follows.

Impairment in Orthosympathetic System

Orthosympathetic centers are present in the spinal lateral column between thoracic 1 and lumbar 2 and cardiac control mainly arises from tract T1-T6 . Thus a lesion above T6 reduces the possibility of increasing heart rate (HR) and cardiac contractility (CC). In tetraplegic patients the orthosympathetic control of the heart is completely abolished and only vagal fibres link encephalic centers to the heart. Therefore, there is no possibility of increasing HR and CC except by reducing vagal heart inhibition. The maximum HR that can be attained in this case is the spontaneous auto-excitatory rate of synousal pacemaker cells, i.e. 100-120 beats min^{-1}. When the lesion is below T6 the possibility of increasing HR and CC is the same as in able bodied persons (i.e. 220 minus the age in years). If the lesion affects the thoracic spinal cord, the sympathetic control of the splancnic vascular district is impaired and the ability to drive the blood contained in this district (in venous capacitance vessels) to fill the heart chambers is reduced. Furthermore, the deficiency in renal sympathetic control reduces the possibility of activating the Renin-Angiotensin system. It must be remembered that Angiotensins II and III exert their action both on vascular walls, increasing muscular tone, and on the heart, so increasing CC. Also, the sympathetic control of surrenalic glands can be lost. In this case surrenalic epynephrine hormone cannot be activated.

The thermoregulatory control of the cutaneous vascular district and sweat glands in the lower part of the body is impaired because of the interruption of the descending pathway from diencephalic thermostatic to sympathetic spinal centers. Thus, in thermal stress the heat dissipation mechanism of vasodilatation and sweating in the lower body is lost. Furthermore, the interruption of the spinothalamic tract, which conveys information from cutaneous thermoreceptors, reduces the ability to maintain thermal homeostasis. This fact is reflected in the shiver paradox: when the lower part of the body is refrigerated the diencephalic centre, which perceives this manoeuvre because the blood is cool, reacts by shivering. But the subject who is not aware of the cold, due to the interruption of the spinothalamic lateral tract, is surprised by the shivering which is subjectively felt as a purposeless activity. The reduced capacity to be consciously informed about thermal stress can expose the WPA to heat stroke when heavy exercise is performed in hot and humid environments.

Deficiency in Muscular Pump

Hopman et al. [1] have demonstrated that during arm exercise the leg blood volume does not decrease in paraplegic patients, i.e. the patients, unlike able bodied subjects, are not able to redistribute the blood contained in the leg venous mesh. The lack of a muscular blood pump in the paralysed limbs has been indicated as the principal cause of this impairment, even if two other factors can contribute to it: a) the inefficiency of sympathetic output to the lower limb vascular system, which is thus unable to raise the venous wall tone, and b) the reduced capacity of the limb vascular bed.

WPA vs. AA Vascular Adjustment

The above mentioned impairments in WPAs cause a reduction in cardiac efficiency that has been demonstrated by Hopman et al. (see Fig. 2).

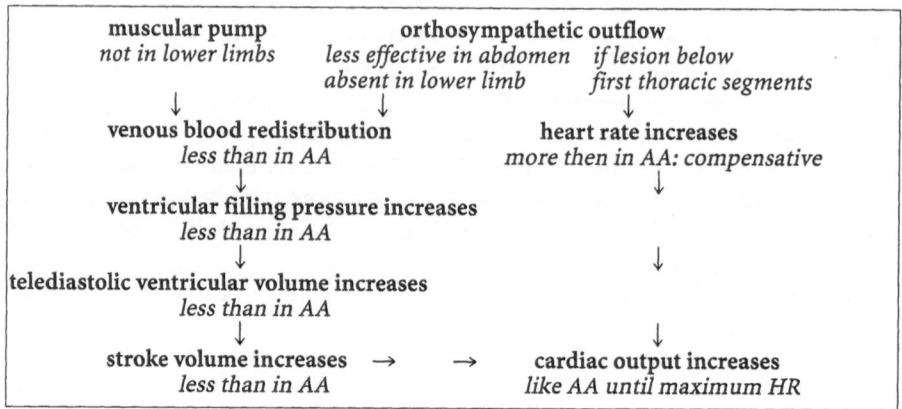

Fig. 2. WPA vs AA: differences in cardiovascular adjustment to exercise

During exercise the reduced possibility of mobilising the blood pooled in the lower body and, consequently the reduced Starling effect, determine a lower stroke volume increment in WPAs than in AAs A WPA with lesion below the first thoracic spinal segments compensates this fact with an increase in HR which at the same oxygen intake ($\dot{V}O_2$) is greater than that in AA. If the exercise is submaximal, at the same O_2 the cardiac output in a WPA is the same as in an AA. When the exercise approximates maximum, HR and cardiac output can not be further increased in a WPA, and the so called hypokinetic circulation starts. If the cardiac output increment does not parallel the $\dot{V}O_2$ increment, only a greater O_2 arterio-venous difference can guarantee an adequate O_2 supply to the muscles.

On-Field Cardiovascular Adjustment in WPA

The cardiovascular adjustment produced by WPAs during actual sports performance has not been directly measured because of the obvious technical difficulties.

Table 1. Cn-field cardiovascular adjustement

Sport	HR (beats · min⁻¹)	%HRmax	$\dot{V}O_2$ (l · min⁻¹)	% $\dot{V}O_2$max
Marathon	175 ± 2	91	2.28+.05	81
Basketball	149 ± 13	79	1.89 +.13	75

The only reliable data we can obtain in this situation are HR and data correlated with energy intake, namely $\dot{V}O_2$, pulmonary ventilation (E) and carbon dioxide production ($\dot{V}CO_2$). It is assumed that at the same percentage of maximal aerobic energy intake ($\dot{V}O_2max$) the cardiovascular adjustments produced on the field are similar to those measured in the laboratory. The values observed during competition in top level paraplegic athletes are reported in table 1. $\dot{V}O_2$, $\dot{V}E$, HR and $\dot{V}CO_2$ were measured in the same subjects during ergometric tests up to exhaustion. It is evident that performing the most demanding sports like marathon or basketball entails energy intake close to $\dot{V}O_2max$. Adopting the linear correlation between cardiac output and $\dot{V}O_2$ calculated by Hopman et al., we could assume that more than 16 l min^{-1} would be pumped by each ventricle in this condition. In Fig 3 a typical trend of a phase of an actual basketball game is presented to show that the energy intake often exceeds the anaerobic threshold. From the trainer's point of view this fact assumes great relevance.

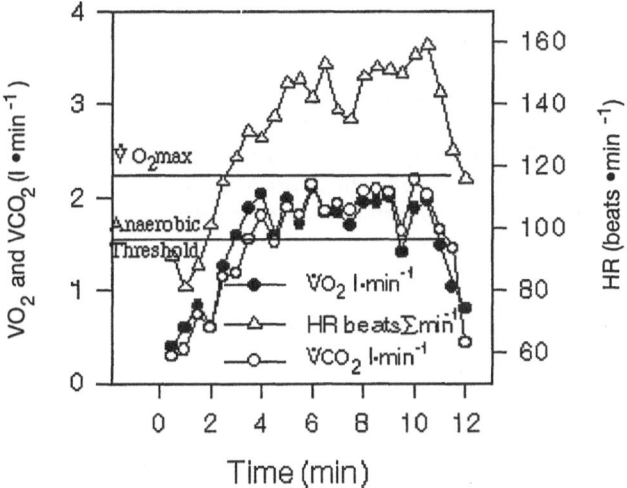

Fig. 3. Tipical trend of a basketball game

Testing WPA Physical Fitness

Data obtained during actual competition are useful in designing an exercise test for health screening in WPAs. Although wheelchair ergometers have the advantage of imitating the on field task, the arm-crank ergometer is the most common device for arm-testing and therefore we have adopted it. The test we adopted is a continuos incremental test with a 20 Watt increment step every 2 minutes until exhaustion. Although ECG is continuously recorded, it is suggested to take a 5 second interruption from the exercise between each step in order to record an ECG trace without EMG artefacts.

On the basis of our experience (more than 70 wheelchair athletes) the linear correlation between HR and $\dot{V}O_2$ was confirmed. Only when the WPA is able to perform the test at least up to 100 Watt (60 Watt for women) the HR reaches values comparable with the maximal theoretical HR and the test is sufficiently provocative to evaluate the eligibility to practice agonistic sport. Another criterion for judging athletic fitness is that 2 minutes after the end of the exercise the HR in young people should be lower than 140 beats min[-1]. These criteria do not apply to patients with lesions at the level of the first thoracic tract who cannot substantially increase the HR because of the deficiency in sympathetic heart control

References

1. Hopman MTE (1994) Circulatory responses during arm exercise in individuals with paraplegia. Int. J. Sport Med,15:126-131
2. Shephard RJ (1988) Sports Medicine and the Wheelchair Athlete. Sport Med, 4:226-247
3. Gutman L (1976) Sport in the Rehabilitation of Spinal Paraplegics and Tetraplegics. Handbook of Clinical Neurology. Ch 29;521-540 Vinken PJ and Bruyn GW (ed) Northern Publishing Company, Amsterdam
4. Jonson RH (1976) Temperature regulation in Spinal Cord Injuries. Ch 21 in Handbook of Clinical Neurology. Vinken P.J and Bruyn GW (Ed)
5. Marchetti M et al (1992) Idoneità allo Sport Agonistico per Atleti su Sedia a Ruote. Quaderni del Centro di Riabilitazione Neuromotoria S. Lucia, 6:1-144

Determinants and Physiological Limits of Cardiac Morphologic Adaptation in Elite Athletes

A. Pelliccia, A. Spataro, F. M. Di Paolo

Institute of Sport Sciences, Department of Medicine, Rome, Italy

Morphologic cardiac adaptation induced by athletic conditioning (athlete's heart) has been recognized since the late century and to date, a large number of studies have described the morphologic features of the hearts of a variety of athletes engaged in different athletic disciplines [1-11]. However, some aspects of athlete's heart are still topics of scientific interest, such as the physiological limits of morphological changes and the criteria of its differentiation from cardiovascular disease [12].

Definition of the physiological limits of athlete's heart has been difficult so far, because most previous studies were based on relatively small populations of athletes, largely confined to men participating in only a limited number of disciplines. Furthermore, in these studies the effect of training in a specific discipline was not evaluated separately from the effect of "constitutional" factors affecting cardiac dimensions, such as body size, gender and age [13-15], which may be varying greatly between athletes. We have had the opportunity to evaluate the role of these different determinants in a large population of almost 1000 highly trained Italian male and female athletes, separately assessing the impact of type of sport, body surface area, gender and age by applying a multivariate statistical analysis [16]. The results of this study showed that: a) type of sport was an independent determinant of cardiac dimensions, and b) constitutional factors explained about 50% of the variability of cardiac dimensions in athletes, with body surface area being associated with most of this variability.

Effect of Type of Sport

Different athletic disciplines may have very different impacts on cardiac dimensions (Fig. 1), with endurance disciplines being associated with the greatest increase of left ventricular dimensions [16]. Highly trained athletes engaged in cycling, rowing, canoeing and swimming show the largest absolute left ventricular cavity dimensions and wall thickness among elite athletes [17]. Furthermore, in longitudinal studies performed at different times of the training program, substantial changes of left ventricular cavity dimension and/or wall thickness have been found, again mostly in endurance athletes [18-20].

Athletes engaged in power disciplines, such as weight-lifting show relatively larger changes in left ventricular walls thickness than in cavity size. Training in

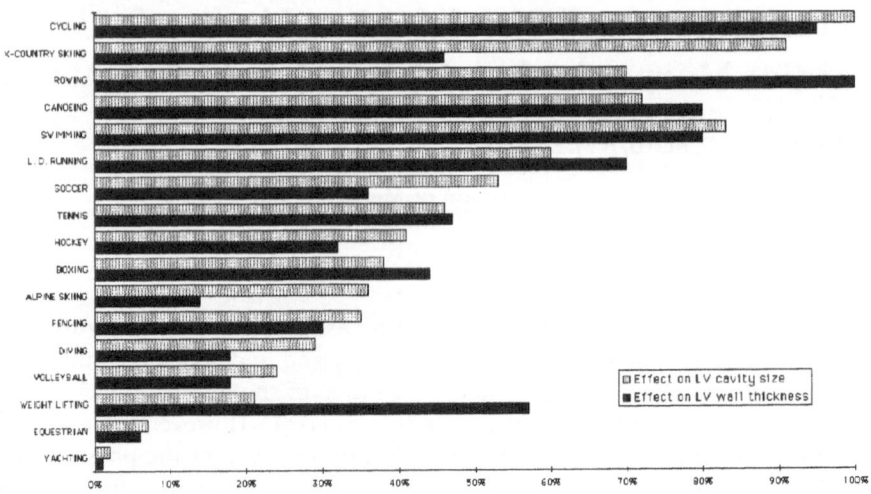

Fig. 1. Effects of different types of sport on left ventricular cavity dimension (*grey bars*) and wall thickness (*block bars*) as percentage of maximum (Derived from results of study [16])

such disciplines is associated with mild absolute wall thickening which, however, does not usually exceed the upper normal limits (ie., 12 mm) [21].

Team training and ball disciplines such as soccer, and volleyball, field hockey water polo, are associated with a moderate and relatively balanced impact on left ventricular cavity dimensions and wall thickness. Absolute left ventricular dimensions are increased in these athletes, but wall thickness usually remains within normal limits, whereas left ventricular cavity dimension is only occasionally enlarged to $\geq$ 60 mm [16].

Finally, participation in technical disciplines, such as equestrian sports or yachting, is associated with virtually no effect on left ventricular dimensions [16].

Hemodynamic overload is generally regarded as the principal physiologic mechanism by which athletic training may modify cardiac dimensions. Hemodynamic overload is different in various types of exercise: in high intensity endurance exercise cardiac output may increase to 35 l/min or more [22] and peak systolic blood pressure may reach 200 mmHg or more [23]. Therefore, athletes engaged in endurance disciplines undergo a pressure and volume overload that usually exceeds in intensity and duration that observed in other disciplines, and eventually induces the most evident left ventricular cavity enlargement and wall thickening.

Training in purely power disciplines is associated with peak systolic blood pressures of 300 mmHg or more and diastolic pressures of 200 mmHg or more [24, 25]. However, the overall period of pressure overload is of limited duration in training sessions and morphologic changes in these athletes are almost confined to a mild wall thickening, while left ventricular cavity size is not significantly altered.

In disciplines such as soccer and other team games, alternate phases of intensive muscular work and recovery occur and periodic increases of cardiac output and blood pressure are sustained [26]. As a result left ventricular dimensions increase in these athletes, but absolute changes are usually of limited extent with a prevalent enlargement of left ventricular cavity dimension.

Finally, no significant hemodynamic overload occurs in purely technical disciplines [27] and no cardiac morphologic changes are usually found in athletes participating in these activities.

Effect of Costitutional Factors

a) **Body size.** Several studies have shown that cardiac dimensions are strictly related to body size [14, 15, 28, 29] and regression equations for calculation of 95% prediction interval of cardiac dimensions as a function of age and body weight have been established [15]. In our athlete population, body surface area proved to be the strongest constitutional determinant of cardiac dimensions and was associated with most of the inter-individual differences related to constitutional factors [16].

b) **Gender.** Recently, there has been growing interest in evaluating the effect of gender on cardiac adaptation to athletic training. Most previous studies were largely confined to men and so information on cardiac morphologic adaptation in women is relatively scarce [9]. Longitudinal studies in women engaged in endurance training have described a 2% to 7% enlargement of left ventricular cavity and a wall thickening of 4% to 12% [30-32]. Recently, we had the opportunity to evaluate a large population of 600 highly trained women athletes participating in a total of 27 different disciplines [33]. Of the women, those engaged in endurance sports, such as cycling, rowing, canoeing and cross country skiing showed the largest increase of left ventricular dimensions, as was previously reported in men [16, 17]. In comparison to men, however, women athletes show smaller absolute left ventricular cavity dimension and wall thickness, probably as a result of several determinants, including lower body size and lean body mass [13, 14, 29], as well as a lower absolute increase of cardiac output and blood pressure during exercise [34-37].

c) **Age.** Aging is also an independent determinant of cardiac dimensions in athletes [13,16]. It has been shown that senior endurance athletes usually have cardiac dimensions greater than junior teammates engaged in the same discipline [38]. Indeed, the best performances are usually achieved by these athletes in their 30s. The increased cardiac dimensions in senior athletes are probably in relation to their larger body surface area and lean body mass, but also to the longer duration of intensive athletic conditioning.

d) Finally, a **genetic control** is suggested by studies evaluating aerobic per-formance and cardiac dimensions in series of twins [39 ,40]. Inherited factors may have a role in governing cardiac dimensions in athletes, either by regulat-ing cardiac morphologic adaptations to training, or through a predisposition to sustain a more intensive athletic conditioning and hemodynamic overload.

Physiological Limits of Morphologic Cardiac Adaptation

In the vast majority of highly trained athletes absolute values of cardiac dimensions are within the accepted normal limits and no question of differential diagnosis with cardiac disease is usually raised. In fact, in a review of echocardiographic studies including almost 800 athletes, the average increase did not exceed 10% for left ventricular cavity dimension, and about 15% for left ventricular thickness in athletes compared to untrained controls [9].

However, in a subset of elite athletes (about 2%), mostly those engaged in rowing and canoeing, absolute left ventricular wall thickening exceeds the normal limit of 12 mm and may reach up to 16 mm, which likely represents the upper limit of physiological wall thickening [17]. Constitutional traits of these athletes are large body surface area and male gender. Furthermore, this subset of athletes is characterized by long term training and competitions at international level, with relevant achievements in World Championships and Olympic Games. The morphologic features of athlete's heart may resemble, in such circumstances, those of hypertrophic cardiomyopathy. Criteria for distinguishing this extreme physiological wall thickening from that of hypertrophic cardiomyopathy have been recently and extensively reviewed [12].

On the other hand, in a sizeable proportion of elite athletes (about 14%), left ventricular cavity dimension may be enlarged above the normal limits ($\geq$ 55 mm) and transverse end-diastolic dimension, as evaluated by echocardiography, may increase up to 70 mm, which represents the upper limit of physiological enlargement [41]. Usual constitutional traits of these athletes are large body size and male gender, with most of them engaged in aerobic disciplines and primarily cycling, cross country skiing and rowing. In these athletes left ventricular cavity dilatation may resemble that found in patients with idiopathic dilated cardiomyopathy. However, in athletes left ventricular systolic function is consistently normal and allows a differentiation between physiological left ventricular dilatation of athlete's heart and pathological dilatation of idiopathic dilated cardiomyopathy [12].

Finally, since cardiac morphological adaptations are the physiological response to intensive athletic conditioning, dynamic changes of cardiac dimensions occur in athletes in response to variations of training load [18-20]. Therefore, serial echocardiographic studies may show substantially different cardiac dimensions in athletes and may aid in distinguishing morphologic features of athlete's heart from other pathologic conditions [20].

References

1. Morganroth J, Maron BJ, Henry WL, Epstein SE (1975) Comparative left ventricular dimensions in trained athletes. Ann Intern Med 82:521-524
2. Roeske WR, O'Rourke RA, Klein A, Leopold G, Karliner JS (1976) Noninvasive evaluation of ventricular hypertrophy in professional athletes. Circulation 53:286-292
3. Ikaheimo MJ, Palatsi IJ:, Takkunen JT (1979) Noninvasive evaluation of the athletic heart: sprinters versus endurance runners. Am J Cardiol 44:24- 30
4. Longhurst JC, Kelly AR, Gonyea WJ, Mitchell JH (1980) Echocardiographic left ventricular masses in distance runners and weight lifters. J Appl Physiol 48:154- 162
5. Keul J, Dickuth HH, Simon G, Lehmann M (1981) Effect of static and dynamic exercise on heart volume, contractility, and left ventricular dimensions. Circ Res (Suppl I) 48:I-162- I-170
6. Ricci G, Lajoie D, Petitclerc R, Peronnet F, Ferguson R J, Fournier M, Taylor A W (1982) Left ventricular size following endurance, sprint and strength training. Med Sci Sports Exerc 14:344-347
7. Fagard R, Aubert A, Lysens R, Staessen J, Vanhees L, Amery A(1983) Noninvasive assessment of seasonal variations in cardiac structure and function in cyclists. Circulation 67:896- 901
8. Fagard R, Aubert A, Staessen J, Van den Eynde E, Vanhees L, Amery A (1984) Cardiac structure and function in cyclists and runners. Comparative echocardiographic study. Br Heart J 52:124-129
9. Maron BJ (1986) Structural features of the athlete heart as defined by echocardiography. J Am Coll Cardiol 7:190-203
10. Van Den Broeke C, Fagard R (1988) Left ventricular structure and function, assessed by imaging and doppler echocardiography, in athletes engaged in throwing events. Int J Sports Med 9:407-411
11. Fisher AG, Adame TD, Yahowitz FG, Ridges JD, Orsmond G, Nelson AG (1989) Noninvasive evaluation of world class athletes engaged in different modes of training. Am J Cardiol 63:337-341
12. Maron BJ, Pelliccia A, Spirito P (1995) Cardiac disease in young trained athletes: insights into methods for distinguishing athlete's heart from structural heart disease, with particular emphasis on hypertrophic cardiomyopathy. Circulation 91:1596-1601
13. Astrand PO (1956) Human physical fitness with special reference to sex and age. Physiol Rew 36:307-335
14. Gardin JM, Savage DD, Ware JH, Henry WL (1987) Effect of age, sex, body surface area on echocardiographic left ventricular wall mass in normal subjects. Hypertension (Suppl II) 9:II-36- II-39
15. Henry WL, Gardin JM, Ware JH (1980) Echocardiographic measurements in normal subjects from infancy to old age. Circulation 62:1054-1061
16. Spirito P, Pelliccia A, Proschan M, Granata M, Spataro A, Bellone P, Caselli G, Biffi A, Vecchio C, and Maron BJ (1994) Morphology of the "athlete's heart" assessed by echocardiography in 947 elite athletes representing 27 sports. Am J Cardiol 74:802-806
17. Pelliccia A, Maron BJ, Spataro A, Proschan MA, Spirito P(1991) The upper limit of physiologic cardiac hypertrophy in highly trained elite athletes. N Engl J Med 324:295-301
18. Ehsani AA, Hagberg JM, Hickson RC (1978) Rapid changes in left ventricular

dimensions and mass in response to physical conditioning and deconditioning. Am J Cardiol 42:52- 56

19. Martin WHIII, Coyle EF, Bloomfield SA, Enshani AA (1986) Effects of physical deconditioning after intense endurance training on left ventricular dimensions and stroke volume. J Am Coll Cardiol 7:982-989

20. Maron BJ, Pelliccia A, Spataro A, Granata M (1993) Reduction in left ventricular wall thickness after deconditioning in highly trained Olympic athletes. Br Heart J 69:125-128

21. Pelliccia A, Spataro A, Caselli G, and Maron BJ (1993) Absence of left ventricular wall thickening in athletes engaged in intense power training. Am J Cardiol 72:1048-1054

22. Ekblom P, Hermannsen L (1968) Cardiac output in athletes. J Appl Physiol 25:1968-1973

23. Palatini P, Mos L, Di Marco A, Mormino P, Munari L, Del Torre M, Valle F, Pessina AC, Dal Palù C (1987) Intra-arterial blood pressure recording during sports activities. J Hypertens 5 (Suppl 5):479-484

24. MacDougall JD, Tuxen D, Sale DG, Moroz JR, Sutton JR (1985) Arterial blood pressure response to heavy resistance exercise. J Appl Physiol 58:785-790

25. MacDougall JD, McKelvie RS, Moroz DE, Sale DG, McCartney N, Buick F (1992) Factors affecting blood pressure during heavy weight lifting and static contractions. J Appl Physiol 73:1590-1597

26. Tumilty D (1993) Physiological characteristics of elite soccer players. Sports Med 16:80-96

27. Granata M, Danese M, Ziantoni P (1990) Heart rate recording in the riders and horses during training and three-day events official competition. In: Sports, Medicine and Hralth. Proceedings of XXIV World Congress of Sports Medicine. Excerpta Medica. pp 1010-1014

28. Epstein M, Goldberg SJ, Allen HD, Konecke L, Wood J (1975) Great vessels, cardiac chamber and wall growth patterns in normal children. Circulation 67:1124-1129

29. Devereux RB, Lutas EM, Casale PN, Kligfield P, Eisenberg RR, Hammond IW, Miller DH, Reis G, Alderman MH, Laragh JH (1984) Standardization of M-mode echocardiographic left ventricular anatomic measurements. J Am Coll Cardiol 4:1222-1230

30. Lamont LS (1980) Effects of training on echocardiographic dimensions and systolic time intervals in women swimmers. J Sports Med 20:397-404

31. Falsetti H, Gisolfi C, Lemon D, Cohen J, Claxton B, Cramer JA, Lenth RA (1982) Noninvasive evaluation of left ventricular function in trained bicyclists. J Sports Med 22:199-206

32. Crouse SF, Rohack JJ, Jacobsen DJ (1992) Cardiac structure and function in women basketball athletes: seasonal variation and comparisons with nonathletic controls. Res Q Exerc Sports 63:393-401

33. Pelliccia A, Maron BJ, Spataro A, Biffi A, Caselli G, Culasso F (1996) Physiological limits of athlete's heart in women. Jama 276:211-215

34. Zwiren LD, Cureton KJ, Hutchinson P (1983) Comparison of circulatory responses to submaximal exercise in equally trained men and women. Int J Sports Med 4:255-259

35. Higginbotham MB, Morris KG, Coleman E, Cobb R (1984) Sex-related differences in the normal cardiac response to upright exercise. Circulation 70:357-366

36. Mitchell JH, Tate C, Raven P (1992) Acute responses and chronic adaptation to exercise in women. Med Sci Sports Exerc 24 (Suppl):S 258-S 265

37. Gleim GW, Stachenfeld NS, Coplan NL, Nicholas JA (1991) Gender differences in the systolic blood pressure response to exercise. Am Heart J 121:524-530

38. Wieling W, Borghols EAM, Hollander AP, Danner SA, Dunning AJ (1981) Echocardiographic dimensions and maximal oxygen uptake in oarsmen during training. Br Heart J 46:190-195
39. Adams TD, Yanowitz FG, Fisher AG, Ridges JD, Nelson AG, Hagan AD, Williams RR, Hunt SC (1985) Heritability of cardiac size: an echocardiographic and electrocardiographic study of monozygotic and dizygotic twins. Circulation 71:39-44
40. Fagard R, Van Den Broeke C, Bielen E, Amery A (1987) Maximum oxygen uptake and cardiac size and function in twins. Am J Cardiol 60:1362-1367
41. Pelliccia A, Maron BJ, Culasso F, Spataro A, Caselli G (1994) Upper limits of physiologically induced left ventricular cavity enlargement due to athletic training. (Abstr) Circulation 90:I-165

Significance and Prognostic Evaluation of Bradyarrhythmias in Athletes

G. Caselli, R. Ciardo

Institute of Sport Sciences, Department of Medicine, Rome, Italy

Usually the term bradyarrhythmia indicates an arrhythmia producing a stable or intermittent reduction of heart rate.

The electrophysiological mechanisms responsible for these arrhythmias include abnormalities of impulse formation, impulse conduction and combinations of both these mechanisms.

Impulse formation disturbances are due to inhibition of normal sinus node automaticity, resulting varying degrees marked sinus bradycardia or bradyarrythmia, and variably prolonged sinus arrest with or without escaping beats or rhythms.

Abnormalities of impulse propagation or conduction may be localized at different levels of the conduction system, such as the sinus node and perinodal area (sinoatrial blocks), atria and A-V node (A-V blocks of various degrees).

A-V blocks are usually classified into three categories: first degree, second degree (usually subdivided into type I, type II, and high grade or advanced), and third degree (complete). Type I A-V block is almost always due to conduction delay in the A-V node, whereas type II block occurs in or below the bundle of His.

Bradyarrhythmias are observed in highly trained athletes more frequently than in normal untrained subjects. This higher prevalence is attributed to characteristic modifications of the autonomic nervous system following heavy prolonged training, mainly of the endurance type.

Initially it was thought that the changes of neural regulation of the heart were due to an absolute increase in cardiac vagal tone.

Later many authors suggested that endurance training induced decreased influence of cardiac sympathetic tone, with no change or a slight decrease in vagal influence on the pacemaker [1, 6, 8].

Moreover, intensive training also determines by some unknown mechanism, a slowing of the "intrinsic heart rate", often interpreted as a central adaptation mechanism. Many investigations have shown that the intrinsic heart rate decreases after several months of training from a normal mean of 105b/min to a mean of 90b/min [1].

Additional modifications of the sympathetic influence have been decribed at the receptor level. It has been suggested that the decrease in heart rate observed in well trained athletes could be due to a reduced ß-adrenergic receptor activity [7, 13].

Therefore, the difficulty of evaluating the autonomic nervous system of athletes appears evident due to of the complex modifications of the mechanisms of cardiovascular neural regulation induced by training [10].

More recently, the development of a new methodology to study to heart rate variability (HRV) seems to provide a non invasive evaluation of the sympatho-vagal balance modulating the sinoatrial node [9].

In addition to the time domain variables, another interesting technique is that of spectral analysis of the HRV, which provides quantitative markers of sympathetic and vagal control of the sinoatrial node .

Many clinical investigations have been performed using these interesting techniques but there is still disagreement on the results and interpretation of the markers of sympathetic and parasympathetic activities [3-5, 11].

Whatever the mechanism, the decreased influence of cardiac sympathetic tone and the slowing of the intrinsic rate of the S-A node are responsible for the most common bradyarrhythmia found in athletes: the training bradycardia [12].

EKG Holter monitoring has determined the real prevalence of the resting bradycardia produced by exercise training: EKG monitoring that includes sleep and wake periods can show bradycardia in 100% of athletes, 56% of them presenting marked bradycardia (below 40 bpm) with or without atrial or junctional escaping rhythms (Table 1).

Table. 1. Bradyarrhythmias during ambulatory Holter monitoring in 50 top level athletes

Arrhythmias	Athletes n° (% of tot.)	
Sinus bradycardia50	(100%)	
Marked sinus bradycardia	28	(56%)
Sinus pauses > 2 sec.	2	(4%)
Sinus pauses > 3 sec.	–	–
Junctional escaping beats	11	(22%)
Junctional escaping rhythms	6	(12%)
1st degree A-V block	5	(10%)
Type 1, 2nd degree A-V block	2	(4%)

In contrast, athletes rarely show sinus arrest greater than 3 sec or spontaneous sino-atrial blocks. In these cases Holter monitoring is an important diagnostic tool, recording long sinus pauses exclusively during sleep with a normal frequency response of the S-A node during an exercise stress test: this behaviour helps to differentiate the real sinus dysfunction from vagal hypertone (Fig. 1).

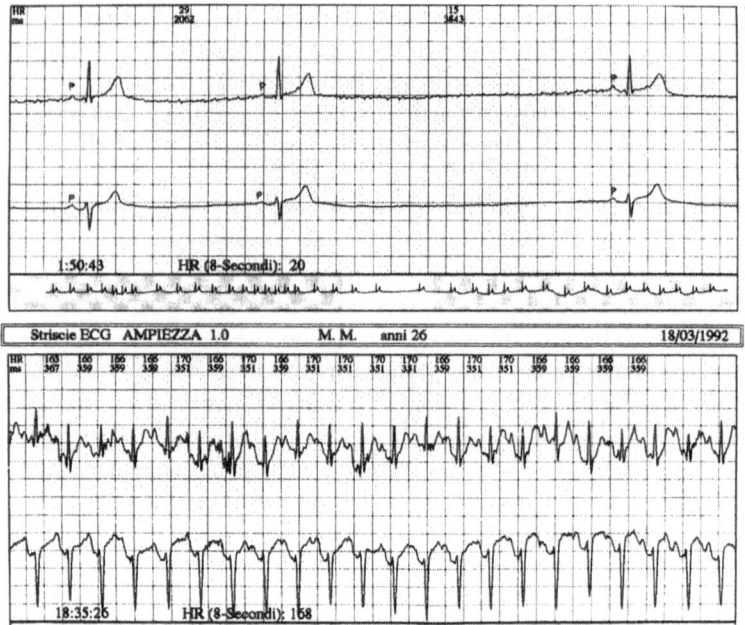

Fig. 1. 26 years old waterpolo player. EKG Holter monitoring showed nocturnal sinus pauses exceeding 3 sec and normal frequency response of the sinus node during training (heart rate near 170 b.p.m.)

However, frequent tests and prolonged follow-up are necessary to exclude a pathologic condition that can lead to a real sinus dysfunction.

The significant prevalence of sinus bradyarrhythmias in athletes is because the relative increase of resting vagal tone following intense physical training is generally predominant at sinus node level. Nevertheless, in some athletes vagal tone may be predominant or selective at A-V node conduction level, so causing the appearance of A-V blocks.

First degree A-V blocks are quite commonly observed in trained athletes, while high degree A-V blocks are a rare finding [2-16]. The prevalence of this phenomenon in athletes during standard EKG varies between 0.15-0.21% and is significantly more frequent than in normal untrained subjects (0.003-0.005%).

In our opinion high degree A-V blocks in athletes are much more frequent than previously reported and the frequent nocturnal occurrence of Wenckenbach phenomena during Holter monitoring in well trained athletes seems to support this (Table 1) [14, 15].

The still controversial problem is whether the relative increase of vagal tone following intensive training may be considered the only factor responsible for the A-V conduction disturbances.

In fact, in addition to the so called functional hypothesis that attributes such

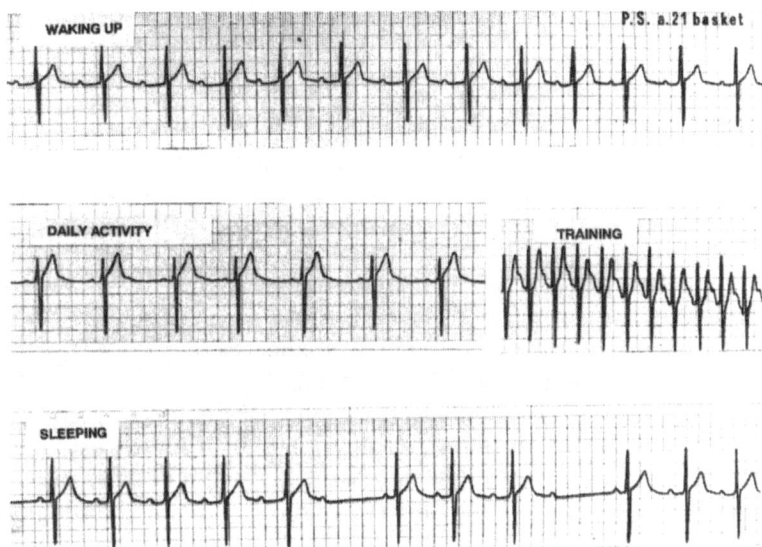

Fig. 2. 21 year old basketball player. EKG Holter monitoring shows the characteristic spontaneous variability of A-V conduction disturbances with the disappearance of A-V block during usual daily activity and training, and the vagally induced worsening of A-V conduction during sleep

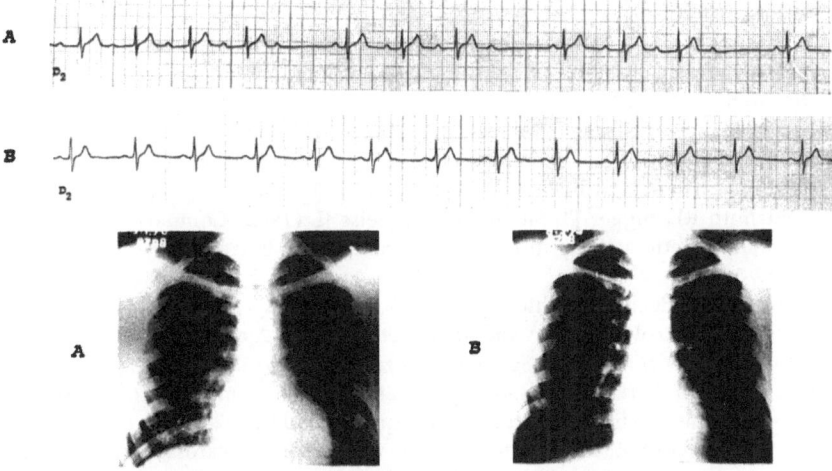

Fig. 3. same case of Fig. 2
Strip A: type 1, 2nd degree A-V block recorded during a period of heavy physical training. Strip B: normal A-V conduction after 1 month of complete detraining. Below: X-Ray before (A) and after detraining (B). After detraining, together with the disappearance of A-V block, a significant reduction in cardiac size was observed

phenomena to a left hemisectorial vagal hypertone with prevalent influence at A-V node level, we cannot ignore the possibility that training may reveal minimal concealed organic alterations of the A-V node.

However, our experience supports the view that A-V block in highly trained athletes must be generally considered as a vagally induced functional phenomenon related to heavy physical training.

This opinion is supported by: a) the disappearance of A-V block during sympathetic stimulation or vagal inhibition and exercise; b) the characteristic spontaneous variability of A-V conduction disturbances during EKG Holter monitoring (Fig. 2); c) the significant correlation of A-V block with the intensity of training (the A-V block is found during intensive physical training and disappears when training is reduced or stopped) (Fig.3); d) the absence of progressive worsening of A-V conduction after a long-term follow-up study [2-16].

The generally benign prognosis of A-V block in clinically asymptomatic athletes must not induce us to ignore the possibility that in a few cases a concealed anomaly of the A-V conduction system may be the cause of high degree A-V blocks, that become evident because of the relative increase of resting vagal tone following heavy physical training.

References

1.   Badeer HS (1984) Cardiovascular Physiology: Neural control of the heart. S. Karger AG Edit. - Basel (Switzerland), pag. 71-80
2.   Caselli G (1984) Significance and prognosis of A-V blocks in athletes. Proceedings of 6° International Congress on Cardiology. The New frontiers of arrhythmias. Marilleva, pag. 393-397
3.   Dixon EM, Kamath MV, Mccartney N, Fallen EL (1992) Neural regulation of heart rate variability in endurance athletes and sedentary controls. Cardiovascular Research 26:713-719
4.   Furlan R, Piazza S, Dell'orto S, Gentile E, Cerutti S, Pagani M, Malliani A (1993) Early and late effects of exercise and athletic training on neural mechanisms controlling heart rate. Cardiovascular Research 27:482-488
5.   Goldsmith RL, Bigger JT, Steinman RC, Fleiss JL (1992) Comparison of 24-hour parasympathetic activity in endurance-trained and untrained young men. JACC 20:552-558
6.   Katona PG, Mclean M, Dighton DH, Guz A (1982) Sympathetic and parasympathetic cardiac control in athletes and nonathletes at rest. J Appl Physiol 52:1652-1657
7.   Lehmann M, Dickhuth HH, Schmid P, Porzig H, Keul J (1984) Plasma catecholamines, ß-adrenergic receptors, and isoproterenol sensitivity in endurance trained and non-endurance trained volunteers. Eur J Appl Physiol 52:362-369
8.   Lin YC, Horvath SM (1972) Autonomic nervous control of cardiac frequency in the exerxise-trained rat. J Appl Physiol 33:796-799
9.   Malliani A, Pagani M, Lombardi F, Cerutti S (1991) Cardiovascular neural regulation explored in the frequency domain. Circulation 84:482-492
10. Mitchell JH (1990) Neural control of the circulation during exercise. Med Sci Sports Exerc 22:141-154
11. Sacknoff DM, Gleim GW, Stachenfeld N, Coplan NL (1994) Effect of athletic trai-

ning on heart rate variability. Am Heart J 127:1275-1278

12. Smith ML, Hudson DL, Graitzer HM, Raven PB (1989) Exercise training bradycardia: the role of autonomic balance. Med Sci Sports Exerc 21:40-44

13. Sylvestre-Gervaise L, Nadeau A, Nguyen MH, Tancrede G, Rousseau-Migneron S (1982) Effects of physical training on ß-adrenergic receptors in rat myocardial tissue. Cardiovascular Research 16:530-534

14. Talan DA (1982) Twenty-four hour continuos ECG recording in long distance runners. Chest 82:19-24

15. Viitasalo MT(1982) Ambulatory electrocardiographic recording in endurance athletes. Br Heart J 47:213

16. Zeppilli P, Fenici R, Sassara M, Pirrami Mm, Caselli G(1980) Wenckebach second-degree A-V block in top ranking athlete: an old problem revisited. Am Heart J 100: 281-294

Prognostic Evaluation of Supraventricular Arrhythmias in Athletes

A. Biffi, G. Piovano, L.Verdile, F. Fernando

Department of Medicine, Institute of Sport Sciences, CONI, Rome, Italy

Supraventricular arrhythmias (SA) affect a large number of subjects. They are generally considered to be benign and are still largely treated by anti arrhythmic drugs. In rare cases and by certain specific mechanisms not only in Wolff-Parkinson-White syndrome (W-P-W), SA may cause sudden cardiac death [1]. Atrial fibrillation is certainly the most common arrhythmia in clinical practice, its prevalence being about 0.2-9% in the adult population, depending on age [2]. However, to date not much is known about the electrophysiologic mechanism of atrial fibrillation, with consequent objective difficulties in defining the vulnerable parameters.

SA are generally classified in three groups:
1) Desynchronised electrical activity-atrial fibrillation (AF).
2) Partially desynchronised electrical activity-atrial fibrillo-flutter
3) Synchronised electrical activity-atrial flutter(AFL) (common and uncommon), atrial tachycardia (AT) and junctional tachycardias (atrio-ventricular nodal re-entry tachycardia-AVNRT and atrio-ventricular re-entry tachycardia due to concealed or evident accessory pathways-AVRT; this latter will not be discussed in this study). After AF, junctional tachycardias are the most frequent arrhythmias in clinical practice.

Recently, radio frequency transcatheter ablation showed its usefulness in the new non-pharmacological treatment of these latter arrhythmias [3]. This electrical approach has to show a favourable risk/benefit ratio in a long-term follow-up before being accepted as first choice/treatment of SA.

SA are often symptomatic for palpitations. Palpitations are not a rare symptom in athletes and, therefore, can worsen physical performance. Unfortunately, the short duration of palpitations often does not allow visualization by surface ECG, exercise stress test or Holter monitoring etc. For this reason, only few reports regarding SA in athletes are available [4, 5]. In an our recent study we assessed the usefulness of transesophageal pacing in identifying SA in athletes symptomatic for palpitations without evidence of cardiac arrhythmias by the standard non invasive diagnostic technique [6]. This study showed the importance of transesophageal atrial pacing particularly when performed at the peak of exercise and during the recovery phase in top-level athletes symptomatic for palpitations during exercise.

Supraventricular Arrhythmias

Atrial Fibrillation

The prevalence of AF or AFL in young competitive athletes is the same as in the general population of the same age. We found a prevalence of AF of 0.2% in our population of 5.000 top-level athletes practising different sports [4]. In particular, in symptomatic arrhythmic athletes AF may be responsible for a high percentage of episodes and it may disturb a professional career. Different studies have shown a prevalence of AF/AFL of 25-40% in symptomatic athletes [4, 6]. This arrhythmia is very easy to reinduce by transesophageal pacing at rest or during exercise and often shows a short duration (Fig. 1). In these athletes, it is very important to exclude the presence of an underlying heart substrate (myocarditis) or metabolic disease (hyperthyroidism) and of W-P-W syndrome. In fact, the electrophysiologic properties of the accessory pathway can accelerate the ventricular rates and increase the probability of degeneration into ventricular fibrillation, especially during physical activity or emotional stress [7]. In athletes, idiopathic AF may be due to a "vagal" or "adrenergic" mechanism, as described by Coumel [8]. The increase of the adrenergic tone caused by physical effort can explain the induction of AF/AFL in some athletes for a variable alteration of atrial refractoriness [9]. Vice versa, the neuro-hormonal imbalance related to prolonged athletic training and resulting in an enhanced vagal tone [10] could also explain the induction of AF at rest or during sleep in other symptomatic athletes. Some authors have shown the disappearance of paroxysmal episodes of AF following athletic detraining for an adequate period of time (mean 20 months) [4]. These data support the hypothesis of a transient unknown myocardial substrate (like myocarditis) as the origin of the arrhythmia [11].

The various and complex electrophysiologic mechanisms of AF make its management difficult: infact, class 1C drugs propafenone and flecainide have been found very effective in slopping an acute AF [12], but show limited efficacy in terms of prophylaxis of arrhythmia recurrences [13].

Atrial Tachycardia

AT is present if the tachycardia rate is regular, the atrio-ventricular conduction is > 1:1 (2:1, 3:1 and so forth) and the atrial rate < 250 beats/minute [14]. On the basis of the electrophysiologic mechanism, AT is divided into automatic, sinus or intraatrial re-entry and triggered forms. Automatic AT can occur in incessant tachycardia. In our high-level athlete population AT was found in 6.2% of the symptomatic athletes (Fig. 1).

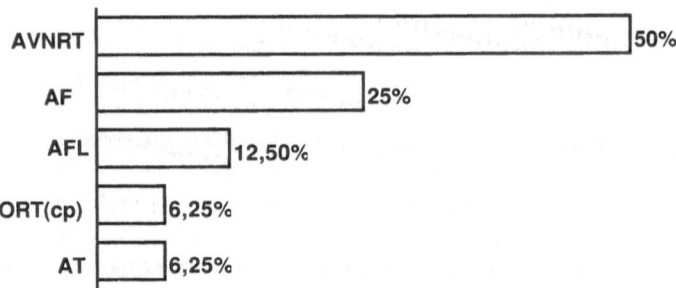

Fig. 1. Supraventricular arrhythmias induced by trans-esophageal pacing in symptomatic top-level athletes AVNRT: AV nodal reentry tachycardia; AF: atrial fibrillation; AFL: atrial flutter; ORT (cp): orthodromic reciprocanting tachycardia (concealed pathway); AT: automatic atrial tachycardia

Junctional Tachycardia (Atrio-ventricular nodal re-entry tachycardia)

AVNRT is a very common SA. In top-level symptomatic athletes AVNRT was responsible for 50% of palpitations (Fig. 1).The re-entry circuit is represented by a slow pathway (with a short refractory period) and a fast pathway (with a longer refractory period) [15]. Usually, the AVNRT goes along the slow pathway in an anterograde way and the fast pathway in retrograde. It is not entirely known that the re-entry circuit be entirely located inside the atrio-ventricular node or include a part of septal atrium [16]. AVNRT showed the greatest inducibility at transesophageal pacing, in particular during exercise [6].

Transesophageal pacing allowed the elucidation of the electrophysiologic mechanism of arrhythmia in many cases and, therefore, has assured a more accurate prognostic evaluation for eventual therapy [17]. The greater inducibility of AVNRT during exercise in athletes with palpitations during exercise could be explained by the influence of the adrenergic tone on the re-entrant circuits. In fact, it has been shown that during exercise the atrio-ventricular node refractoriness and the anterograde pathway of the re-entrant circuits shortens, while the retrograde pathway remains unvaried [18]. This physiologic situation can facilitate the induction of junctional tachycardias [19] by means of an previously described extra stimuli protocol [6]. Furthermore, the enhanced vagal tone, which is a common finding in well-trained athletes, probably reduces the possibility of induction of junctional tachycardias at rest because of the depression of cell action potentials and atrio-ventricular conduction [20]. The duration of AVNRT is generally short and the interruption of the exercise is frequently sufficient to stop the arrhythmia. When AVNRT does not stop spontaneously, an intravenous bolus of propafenone (2 mg/Kg) is very effective [6]. The AVNRT has an excellent prognosis and the pharmacological treatment directed at preventing SA is useful and associated with a good prognosis in follow-up [1].

Unfortunately, young top-level athletes are not ideal patients for a chronic and preventive pharmacological treatment. For the more symptomatic athletes radio frequency ablation represents a major advance in the treatment of SA when compared with surgery, antitachycardia pacemakers or long-term anti-arrhythmic drug treatment [21]. When sufficient electrophysiologic expertise is present success rates above 90% have been noted for a single session of trans-catheter ablation (Table 1).

Table 1. Transcatheter ablation of atrio-ventricular nodal reentry tachycardia (AVNRT)

Authors	Percentage of success		Complications	
	Fast	Slow	Fast	Slow
Lee [22]	82	—	3/39	—
Jazayeri [23]	100	97	4/19	0/35
Wu [24]	100	100	0/10	0/16
Jackman [25]	—	98	—	1/80
Haissaguerre [26]	—	100	—	0/64
Kay [27]	100	88	1/4	0/34

References

1. Wang Y, Scheinman MM, Chien WW et al (1991) Patients with supraventricular tachycardia presenting with aborted sudden death: mechanism and long-term fol-low-up. J. Am Coll Cardiol 18:1711
2. Kannel WB, Wolf PA (1992) Epidemiology of atrial fibrillation. In: Falk RH, Podrid PJ (eds) Atrial Fibrillation: Mechanisms and Management. New York, Raven Press Ltd. 81
3. Gallagher JJ, Svenson RH, Kasell JH et al (1982) Catheter technique for closed-chest ablation of the atrio-ventricular conduction system. N Engl J Med 306:194
4. Furlanello F, Bertoldi A, Dallago M et al (1994) Atrial fibrillation in top-level athle-tes. In Olsson SB, Allessie MA, Campbell RWF (eds) Atrial Fibrillation: mechanisms and therapeutic strategies. Futura Publishing Co Inc, Armonk, NY
5. Delise P, Bonso A, Coro' L et al (1992) Electrophysiologic substrates of idiopathic atrial fibrillation in the general population and in athletes. New Trends Arrhyth 8:719
6. Biffi A, Ammirati F, Caselli G et al (1993) Usefulness of transesophageal pacing during exercise for evaluating palpitations in top-level athletes. Am J Cardiol 72:922
7. Timmermans C, Smeets J, Rodriguez LM et al (1995) Aborted sudden death in the Wolff-Parkinson-White syndrome. Am J Cardiol 76:492.
8. Coumel P, Attuel P, Lavallee JP et al (1978) Syndrome d'arythmie auriculaire d'ori-gine vagale. Arch Mal Coeur 71:645
9. Zipes DP, Mihalick MJ, Robbins GT (1974) Effects of selective vagal and stellate ganglion stimulation on atrial refractoriness. Cardiovasc Res 8:647
10. Badeer HS (1980) Cardiovascular adaptations in the trained athlete. In: Lubich T, Venerando A. (eds) Proceedings of the International Conference on Sports

Cardiology, Rome 1978, Gaggi Bologna, p 3
11. Zeppilli P, Frustaci A (1993) Utilita', limiti ed indicazioni della biopsia miocardica negli sportivi. Int J Sports Cardiol 2:275
12. Crijns HJGM, Van Vijk M, Van Gilst WH et al (1988) Acute conversion of atrial fibrillation to sinus rhythm: clinical efficacy of flecainide acetate. Comparison of two regimens. Eur Heart J 9:634
13. Pritchett ELC, McCarthy EA, Wilkinson WE (1991) Propafenone treatment of symptomatic paroxysmal supraventricular arhhythmias. Ann Inter Med 114:539
14. Waldo AL (1987) Mechanism of atrial fibrillation, atrial flutter and ectopic atrial tachycardia: a brief review. Circulation 75:37
15. Josephson ME (1993) Clinical cardiac electrophysiology. Lea and Febiger, 182
16. Scheinman MM (1985) Atrioventricular nodal or atriojunctional reentrant tachycardia. J Am Coll Cardiol 6:1393
17. Santini M, Ansalone G, Cacciatore G, Turitto G (1990) Transesophageal pacing. PACE 13:1298
18. Deliŝe P, D'Este D, Bonso A et al (1989) Utilità dello studio elettrofisologico transesofageo durante test ergometrico nella valutazione delle tachicardie parossistiche sopraventricolari insorgenti sotto sforzo. G Ital Cardiol 19:1094
19. Brembilla-Perrot B, Terrier de la Chaise A, Pichene M et al (1989) Isoprenaline as an aid to the conduction of the catecholamine-dependent supraventricular tachycardias. Br Heart J 61:348
20. Mazgalev T, Dreifus LS, Michelson EL et al (1986) Vagally induced hyperpolarization in atrioventricular node. Am J Physiol 251:H631-H643
21. Kuck KH, Schluter M (1994) Junctional tachycardia and the role of catheter ablation. Lancet 8857:1386
22. Lee MA, Morady F, Kadish A et al (1991) Catheter modification of the atrioventricular junction with radiofrequncy energy for control of atrioventricular nodal reentry tachycardia. Circulation 83:827
23. Jazayeri Mr, Hempe SL, Sra JS et al (1992) Selective transcatheter ablation of the fast and slow pathways using radiofrequency energy in patients with atrioventricular nodal reentry tachycardia. Circulation 85:1318
24. Wu D, Yeh SJ, Wang CC et al (1992) Nature of dual atrioventricular node pathways and the tachycardia circuit as defined by radiofrequency ablation technique. J Am Coll Cardiol 20:884
25. Jackman WM, Beckman KJ, McClelland JH et al (1992) Treatment of supraventricular tachycardia due to atrioventricular nodal reentry tachycardia by radiofrequency ablation of slow-pathway conduction. N Engl J Med 327:313
26. Haissaguerre M, Gaita F, Fischer B et al (1992) Elimination of atrioventricular nodal reentry tachycardia using discrete slow potentials to guide application of radiofrequency energy. Circulation 85:2162
27. Kay GN, Epstein AE, Dailey et al (1992) Selective radiofrequency ablation of the slow pathway for the treatment of atrioventricular nodal reentry tachycardia: evidence for involvement of perinodal myocardium with the reentrant circuit. Circulation 85:1675

Prognostic Evaluation of Ventricular Arrhythmias in Athletes

G. Ansalone, A. Biffi[1], A. Auriti, B. Magris, M. Santini

Department of Heart Diseases S. Filippo Neri Hospital,
[1]Institute of Sport Sciences, Dept. of Medicine, Rome, Italy

Prevalence of Ventricular Arrhythmias in Normal Subjects

Ventricular arrhythmias (VA) can occur in a variety of heart diseases as well as in normal persons. Although the normal range of the VA is still under debate, there is general agreement that frequent and or complex VA are an uncommon finding in normal subjects without any apparent structural heart disease. Therefore, some degree of VA very likely represents a marker of a pathological condition requiring accurate diagnostic assessment to determine the real impact of the VA in the clinical setting and its preventive and/or therapeutic implications. Generally, the normal range of VA varies from 10 to 100 ventricular premature ectopic beats (VPB) / 24 hour, whereas the complex forms (couplets, multiplets and non-sustained ventricular tachycardia) are usually absent in normal subjects. Non-sustained ventricular tachycardia (NSVT) of more than 10-15 beats, with a rate >150 min., as well as sustained monomorphic or polymorphic ventricular tachycardia (SVT) should also be considered as malignant forms in healthy subjects without evident cardiovascular abnormalities. In fact, idiopathic ventricular tachyarrhythmia is not particularly rare cause of sudden cardiac death, ranging in the literature from 1% to 14% of patients less than 40 years old who have survived an episode of sudden unexpected cardiac arrest [1, 2].

Ventricular Arrhythmias and Risk of Sudden Death

Some earlier studies suggested that ventricular premature beats (VPB), even in apparently healthy persons, were associated with an increased risk of sudden death and an increased incidence of ischemic heart disease [3], whereas more recent studies have suggested that the presence of VPB in apparently healthy persons is not associated with an increased risk of death [4].

According to the Framingham Heart Study [5], the incidental detection of VA may be associated with a two-fold increase in the risk of all-cause mortality and myocardial infarction or death due to coronary heart disease. Consequently, complex or frequent VA may be a marker for occult coronary heart disease or silent ischemia. However, a strong correlation between arrhythmias and outcome was not found even in patients with coronary artery disease. Thus, it is possible that a non-ischemic mechanism underlies arrhythmias and increased risk of cardiac death in men with no clinically apparent coronary heart disease. Many authors [6-9] have suggested that hypertensive subjects may be at increased risk for fatal cardiac events, perhaps because of an increased frequency of ventricular premature beats. In a multivariate model [10, 11] which includes left ventricular hypertrophy and increased left ventricular mass, the VA maintain their significance as an independent risk factor, suggesting that they are not merely a marker for occult left ventricular dysfunction. On the other hand, other studies [12] showed an increased risk of total and sudden mortality in patients with left ventricular hypertrophy and an increased incidence of coronary artery disease in patients with increased left ventricular mass [13, 14]. VA probably represents the fatal link between an increased left ventricular mass as expression of left ventricular hypertrophy and a coronary artery disease in hypertensives, but the real mechanism of this interaction is still unclear. If this mechanism is clarified, another step forward could also be made in our knowledge of the relationship between the physiological increase of left ventricular mass and the complex or frequent VA in athletes. On the whole, in our opinion, it is unlikely that VA per se can become a main pathogenetic factor of SD in healthy persons.

Sudden Death in Apparently Healthy Subjects

Sudden arrhythmic death is rare in the absence of overt heart disease. Previous investigations [15-19] demonstrated that the underlying disease is usually a clinically silent cardiovascular disorder that may not have been diagnosed or even suspected when the victim was alive. Ventricular fibrillation is involved in 80-90% of sudden cardiac death events with coronary artery disease usually the underlying abnormality, but other aetiologies such as cardiomyopathy, valvular heart disease and the long QT syndrome are less common but still well-known causes of ventricular fibrillation. Structural heart disease is absent in up to 5% of survivors of out-of-hospital cardiac arrest [20, 21]. Moreover, 10% to 17% of forensic examinations fail to reveal the cause of sudden death in victims younger than 45 years of age [16, 22, 23]. A review of the world literature on this problem was published by Viskin and Belhassen [2]. Taking 19 studies, they reported a total of 54 patients with a average age of 36 years and a male to female ratio of 2.5 : 1. Over 90% of the patients required resuscitation, with syncope due to non-sustained ventricular fibrillation reported in the remaining patients. Wellens et al. [24] reported nine patients with one or more episodes of circulatory collapse in the absence of overt heart disease or other known causes of arrhythmias. Sudden arrhythmic death occurred in one of these patients 21 months after his first collapse. In eight patients ventricular fibrillation or flutter was documented at the time of resuscitation. The age at the first episode ranged from 16 to 41 years (average 28). The patients were treated with pharmacological therapy and the selection of antiarrhythmic drugs was largely empirical.

Meissner et al. [25] reported 28 survivors of ventricular fibrillation (average age 42 years) with minimal or no structural abnormalities, who were treated with an implantable cardioverter-defibrillator (ICD). During follow-up, an excellent 3-year survival rate was found (there were no cardiac deaths). Particularly, four patients received one "appropriate" shock, suggesting that these patients have a potential risk of recurrent cardiac arrest, fatal outcome of which may be avoided by the ICD discharge.

Sudden Death in Young Competitive Athletes

Maron et al. [26] presented the largest report of 84 cases of sudden death in competitive athletes. Cardiovascular abnormalities were present in 74 (88%). As the causes of "athletic field" deaths, the authors observed: 1) hypertrophic cardiomyopathy (47%), 2) coronary abnormalities (13%), 3) myocarditis (6%), 4) rupture of the aorta (6%) and 5) dilated cardiomyopathy (4%) (Fig. 1). Thus, hypertrophic cardiomyopathy was reported by Maron et al. as the major cause of athlete death.

Corrado et al. [27], studying by postmortem examination 182 young victims (< 35 years) who had died suddenly in the Veneto region (northern Italy) showed that this fatal event was sports-related in 31 and non-sports-related in 151 athletes. The main abnormality found in the sports-related sudden deaths was right ventricular cardiomyopathy (26%), with the other disclosed abnormalities being: coronary atherosclerosis (20%), conduction system pathology (10%), anomalous coronary artery (10%), mitral valve prolapse (6%), hypertrophic cardiomyopathy (3%), myocarditis (3%), aortic dissection (3%), others (19%) (Fig. 2). In this study, regardless of the relation between sudden death

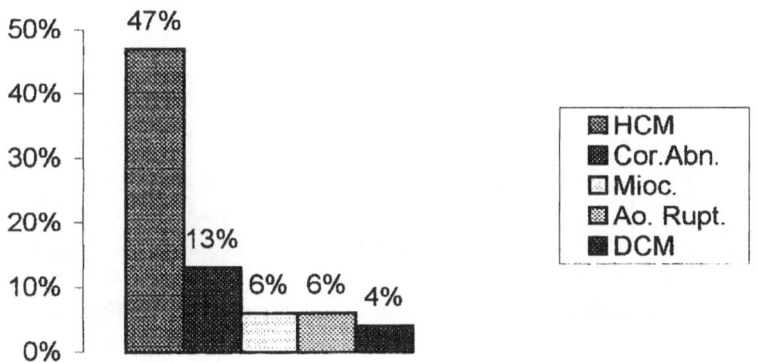

Fig. 1. Causes of athletic death (Mod. by Maron et al. Circ. 1993) (26). HCM: hypertrophic cardiomyopathy. Cor.Abn.: coronary abnormalities. Myoc.: Myocarditis. Ao. Rupt.: aortic rupture. DCM: dilated cardiomyopathy

and sports activity, coronary atherosclerosis became the major cause of death (41%), the right ventricular cardiomyopathy rose to 33%, while hypertrophic cardiomyopathy was present only in the 8% of the dead athletes. The abnormalities that strongly correlated with sports-related deaths were of anomalous coronary artery origin (p< 0.001) and right ventricular cardiomyopathy (p< 0.01). Of all causes of sudden death in patients with minimal structural abnormalities, mitral valve prolapse (MVP) was also emphasized by many authors [28, 29], but today it is well known that only a minority of these subjects are actually exposed to a risk of sudden death: patients with complex VA, hemodynamically significant mitral valve regurgitation, prolonged QT interval, inferolateral repolarization abnormalities, thickened mitral leaflets, history of syncope, presyncope and palpitations. Nishimura et al. [30] found six cases of sudden death among 237 minimally symptomatic patients with MVP followed-up for an average of 6 years, suggesting an annual mortality rate of approximately 40 per 10.000. This is twice the incidence of sudden death expected in the general adult population. All patient victims of sudden death in this report had echocardiographic evidence of mitral leaflet thickening, which was found in 41% of their patients and might represent, besides VA, an important discriminator between subjects with high and low risk. However, two thirds of the cases of sudden death occurred in men older than 55 years of age and, in the absence of autopsy confirmation, an occult ischemic disease could explain this high mortality rate.

On the whole, a dramatic event as sudden death is unlikely to occur in subjects free from any cardiac abnormalities, occuring usually only in people with occult underlying heart diseases.

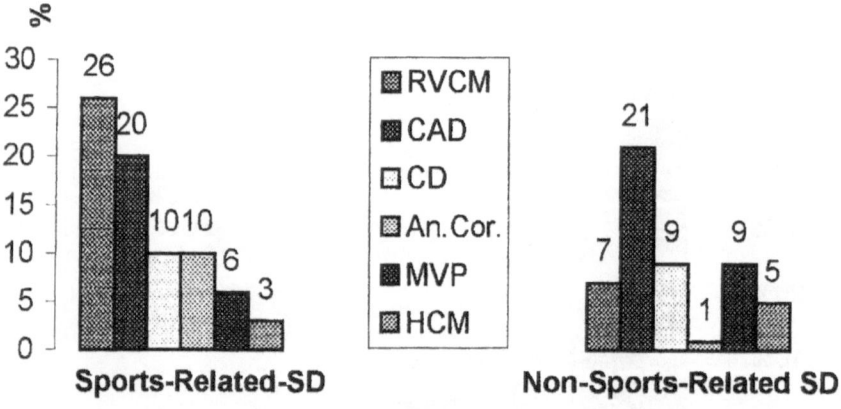

Fig. 2. Causes of sports-related and non-sports-related SD [27]. RVCM: right ventricular cardiomyopathy. CAD: coronary artery disease. CD: conduction disturbances. Cor. An: coronary anomalies. MVP: mitral valve prolapse. HCM: hypertrophic cardiomyopathy

Clinical Aspects of Ventricular Arrhythmias and Prognosis

The prognosis in patients with ventricular tachyarrhythmias without structural heart disease has been described as excellent. However, the prognosis may be less favourable in the subgroup of patients surviving an episode of ventricular fibrillation or flutter. Patients with primary electrical disturbance featuring ventricular fibrillation are at high risk of recurrence of major arrhythmic events during a long-term follow-up [25, 31]. Non-inducibility at baseline electrophysiologic study (EPS) does not predict an uneventful course [24, 25, 31]. Also, early defibrillator implantation should be considered in these patients [25, 31], since selection of antiarrhythmic drug therapy is largely empirical [24]. Sustained monomorphic VT or rapid non-sustained polimorphic VT if hemodynamically well tolerated might have a less unfavourable prognosis than VF but the tendency is to consider also these arrhythmias malignant and as requiring an accurate clinical surveillance together with programmed ventricular stimulation guided pharmacological therapy. Moreover, ICD must be considered in patients unresponsive to drugs. NSVT and complex or frequent VPBs must be considered potentially malignant in patients with coronary atherosclerosis, but usually have a good prognosis in subjects with short and asymptomatic runs and without overt heart disease.

Mechanisms of Ventricular Tachyarrhythmias in Healthy Subjects

As the mechanism of reentry is involved only in a few patients EPS reproducibility on of the arrhythmia is rather low, ranging from 39% [25] to 53% [31]. In others the tachyarrhythmia can be initiated by a short-coupled VPB which usually starts a polimorphic NSVT responsible for syncopal episodes. In the remaining patients one has to consider the possibility that the arrhythmias are caused by early after-depolarizations [24]. Neverthless, the mechanism of the arrhythmia cannot always be accurately defined and remains a subject of speculation. Many subjects with right ventricular cardiomyopathy show frequent or complex VPBs with left bundle branch block morphology, as well as short runs of monomorphic ventricular tachycardia with the same morphology. The presence of this type of arrhythmia makes one suspect a reentrant pathway in the region of altered myocardium of the right ventricular wall.

Diagnostic Evaluation of Ventricular Arrhythmias in Healthy Subjects

Because idiopathic tachyarrhythmia is a diagnosis "by exclusion", considerable effort must be made to rule out underlying heart disease. In asymptomatic or minimally in symptomatic subjects, a non-invasive diagnostic evaluation can suffice, consisting of a careful clinical history, physical examination, 12-lead

ECG, 24-hour Holter monitoring including a training or competitive session if possible, exercise testing with the Bruce protocol and Valsalva manoeuvre, laboratory tests, chest roentgenograms, Doppler hechocardiography, radionuclide assessment of both left and right ventricular performance and signal-averaged ECG. Pre-excitation patterns and long QT interval (corrected by Bazett's formula), either stable or transient, such as metabolic or electrolyte disturbances, must be excluded. An increase of VPBs or the appearance of repetitive arrhythmias during exercise deserve further evaluation. In some of these athletes thought to have a structurally normal heart, cardiac catheterization and angiography may reveal otherwise undetected abnormalities including occult coronary artery disease, congenital coronary anomalies, arrhythmogenic right ventricular dysplasia, cardiac tumor or evidence of cardiomyopathy [32]. On the other hand, in subjects without an increase of VA during exercise, time and frequency domain SAECG is useful to complete the evaluation since the absence of ventricular late potentials has a high negative predictive value for malignant arrhythmias and underlying structural heart disease.

Patients with syncopal episodes thought to be caused by VA should undergo cine-magnetic resonance, cardiac catheterization with angiography of both ventricles, coronary angiography and multiple right ventricular endomyocardial biopsies. EPS with inducibility test is needed in these cases to verify induction of ventricular tachyarrhythmia associated with hemodynamic collapse.

Guidelines for Athletic Participation of Athletes with Ventricular Arrhythmias

According to the Task Force on Arrhythmias of ACC [32] and considering the Italian Cardiologic Committee for Eligibility to Competitive Sports (COCIS), it should be remembered that:

Athletes with complex VPB (Figure 3)
1) Athletes with no structural heart disease, having VPB only at rest or during exercise testing or on Holter monitoring recorded during a training session or competition, usually do not need any drug treatment and can participate in all competitive sports. The same athletes in whom VPB increase during effort, producing symptoms of impaired consciousness and significant fatigue or dyspnea, may participate in low-intensity competitive sports only (class IA).
2) Athletes with structural heart disease and VPB who are in high-risk groups, whether suppressed by drug therapy or not, may participate in low-intensity competitive sports only (class IA).

Athletes with NSVT (Figure 4)
1) Athletes with symptomatic NSVT, or completion of indicated invasive and non-invasive diagnostic procedures, should not compete in any sport for at least 6 months after the last episode of VT, regardless of whether they are treat-

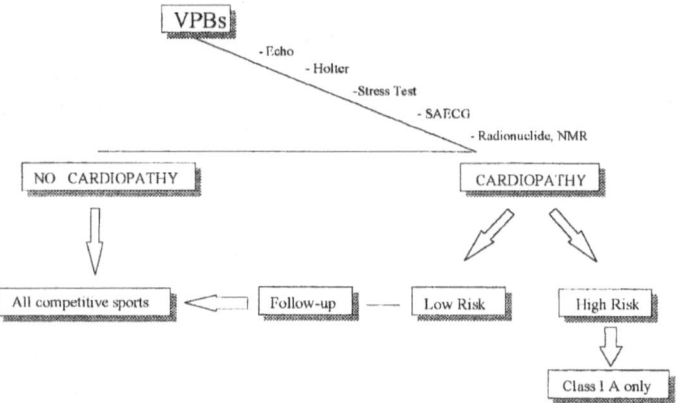

Fig. 3. Decision-making in athletes with complex ventricular premature beats (VPBs). NMR : cine-magnetic resonance. SAECG : signal averaged ecg. Radionuclide : left and right ventricular radionuclide assessment. Class I A : very low dynamic activities (billiards, bowling, cricket, curling, golf, riflery)

ed with pharmacological or non-pharmacological interventions or not. This follow-up period must include a detraining interval.

In athletes without structural heart disease, in the absence of clinical recurrences of the arrhythmia, and if VT is not inducible by exercise testing and EPS, all competitive sports may be permitted.

No sports are allowed in athletes with structural heart disease or those with recurrences of the arrhythmia after the follow-up and detraining period.

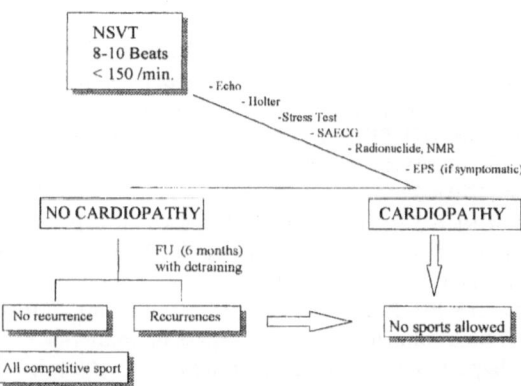

Fig. 4. Decision-making in athletes with non-sustained ventricular tachycardia (NSVT). EPS : electrophysiological study. NMR : cine-magnetic resonance. SAECG : signal averaged ECG. Radionuclide : left and right ventricular radionuclide assessment

Athletes with a pacemaker device

Subjects carrying a pacemaker are not eligible to all moderate and high intensity sports, wheareas low intensity competitive sports (class IA), and also leisure activities not involving a significant risk of trauma to the device can be permitted.

References

1. Cobb LA, Baum RS, Alvarez H III, Schaffer WA (1975) Resuscitation from out-of-hospital ventricular fibrillation: 4 years follow-up. Circulation 51/52 (Suppl III): 223-228
2. Viskin S, Belhassen B (1990) Idiopathic ventricular fibrillation. Am Heart J 120:661-671
3. Rabkin SW, Mathewson FA, Tate RB (1981) Relationship of ventricular ectopy in men'without apparent heart disease to occurrence of hyschemic heart disease and sudden death. Am Heart J 101:135-142
4. Rodstein M, Wolloch L, Gubner RS (1971) Mortality study of the significance of the extrasistoles in an insured population. Circulation 44:617-625
5. Bikkina M, Larson MG, Levy D (1992) Prognostic implications of asymptomatic ventricular arrhythmias: The Framingham Heart Study. Annals of Internal Med 117:990-996
6. Multiple Intervention Trial Research Group (1982) Multiple Risk Factor Intervention Trial risk factor changes and mortality results. JAMA 248:1465-77
7. Medical Council Working Party (1985) MRC trial of treatment of mild hypertension : principal results. Br Med J (Clin Res Ed) 291:97-104
8. Levy D, Anderson KM, Christiansen JC, Campanile G, Stokes J 3d (1988) Antihypertensive drug therapy and arrhythmia risk. Am J Cardiol. 62:147-9
9. The Medical Research Council Working Party on Mild to Moderate Hypertension (1983) Ventricular extrasystoles during thiazide treatment: sub-study of MRC mild hypertension trial. Br Med J 287:1249-53
10. Levy D, Garrison RJ, Savage DD, Kannel WB, Castelli WP (1990) Prognostic implications of echocardiographically determined left ventricular mass in the Framingham Heart Study. N Engl J Med 322:1561-1566
11. Levy D, Anderson KM, Savage DD, Balkus SA, Kannel WB, Castelli WP (1987) Risk of ventricular arrhythmias in left ventricular hypertrophy: the Framingham Heart Study. Am J Cardiol 60:560-565
12. Messerli FH, Ventura HD, Elizardi DJ, Dunn FG, Frolich ED (1984) Hypertension and sudden death. Increased ventricular ectopic activity in left ventricular hypertrophy. Am J Med 77:18-22
13. Levy D, Garrison RJ, Savage DD, Kannel WB, Castelli WP (1989) Left ventricular mass and incidence of coronary heart disease in elderly cohort. The Framingham Heart Study. Ann Intern Med 110:101-107
14. Casale PN, Devereux RB, Milner M, Zullo G, Harshfield GA, Pickering TG (1986) Value of echocardiographic left ventricular mass in predicting cardiovascular morbidity events in hypertensive men. Ann Intern Med 105:173-178
15. Maron BJ, Roberts WC, McAllister MA et al (1980) Sudden death in young athletes. Circulation 62:218-29
16. Topaz O, Edwards JE (1985) Pathologic features of sudden death in children, adolescents, and young adults. Chest 87:476-82

17. Thiene G, Gambino A, Corrado D, Nava A (1986) The pathological spectrum underlying sudden death in athletes. New Trends in Arrhythmias 1:323-331
18. Thiene G., Pennelli N, Rossi L (1983) Cardiac conduction system abnormalities as a possible cause of sudden death in young athletes. Hum Pathol 14:70-74
19. Thiene G, Nava A, Corrado D, Rossi L, Pennelli N (1988) Right ventricular cardiomyopathy and sudden death in young people. N. Engl J Med 318:129-133
20. Wilber DJ, Garan H, Finkelstein D (1988) Out-of-hospital cardiac arrest: use of electrophysiologic testing in the prediction of long-term outcome. N Engl J Med 318: 19-24
21. Myerburg RJ, Kessler KM, Estes D (1984) Long-term survival after prehospital cardiac arrest: analysis of outcome during an 8 year study. Circulation 70:538-546
22. Kramer MR, Drory Y, Lev B (1988) Sudden death in young soldiers: high incidence of syncope prior to death. Chest 93:345-347
23. Philips M, Robinowitz M, Higgins JR, Boran KJ, Reed T, Virmani R (1986) Sudden cardiac death in Air Force recruits: a 20-year review. 256:2696-9
24. Wellens HJJ, Lemery R, Smeets JL, Brugada P, Gorgels AP, Cheriex EC, de Zwaan C (1992) Sudden arrhythmic death without overt heart disease. Circulation 85 (suppl I):I 92-97
25. Meissner MD, Lehmann MH, Steinman RT, Mosteller RD, Akhtar M, Calkins H, Cannom DS, Epstein AE, Fogoros RN, Bing Liem L, Marchlinski FE, Myerburg R, Veltri EP (1993) Ventricular fibrillation in patients without significant structural heart disease: A multicenter experience with implantable cardioverter-dwfibrillator therapy. J Am Coll Cardiol 21:1406-1412
26. Maron BJ, Shirani J, Mueller FO, Cantu RC, Roberts WC (1993) Cardiovascular causes of "athletic field" deaths: analysis of sudden death in 84 competitive athletes (abstr.). Circulation 88 (Suppl I):I-50
27. Corrado D., Thiene G., Nava A., Basso C., Dalla Volta S (1993) Sports-related sudden death in young people (abstr.). Circulation 88, n.4, part II: I-51
28. Winkle RA, Lopes MG, Popp RL, Hancock EW (1976) Life-threatening arrhythmias in yhe mitral valve prolapse syndrome. Am J Med 60:961-7
29. Kligfield P, Levy D, Devereux RB, Savage D (1987) Arrhythmias and sudden death in mitral valve prolapse. Am Heart J 113 (n.5):1298-1307
30. Nishimura RA, McGoon MD, Shub C, Miller FA, Ilstrup DM, Tajik AJ (1985) Echocardiographically documented mitral-valve prolapse. New Engl J Med 313:1305-9
31. Vewer EFD, Hauer RNW, Oomen A, Peters RHJ, Bakker PFA, Robles de Medina EO (1993) Unfavourable outcome in patients with primary electrical disease who survived an episode of ventricular fibrillation. Circulation 88:1021-1029
32. Zipes DP, Garson A (1994) Task Force 6: Arrhythmias. JACC, 24 (n.4):892-899

Radiofrequency Ablation in the Therapy of Wolff-Parkinson-White Syndrome

R. Cappato

II Medical Department, St. Georg Hospital, Hamburg, Germany

Introduction

Successful surgical division of an accessory atrioventricular connection in a patient with Wolff-Parkinson-White syndrome was first reported in 1968 [1]. This ushered in the era of ablative therapy for arrhythmias. The rationale of ablation is that irreversible alteration can be brought on to a discrete anatomical substrate responsible for arrhythmia generation and/or perpetuation.

The next technique using the same rationale was high-voltage direct current catheter ablation [2, 3]. This closed-chest technique overcame the significant morbidity associated with open thoracotomy; however, due to the relatively uncontrolled nature of this energy form which produced thermal, electrical and physical injury (barotrauma), concerns were raised about trauma to thin-walled structures in the heart such as the atrial freewall and the coronary sinus. Alternative modalities were therefore pursued including intracoronary ethanol infusion [4], laser irradiation [5], cryothermy [6], microwave [7], ultrasound [8] and radiofrequency (RF) [9-16] ablation.

With evolving understanding of anatomical-electrophysiological relationships, improvement of mapping techniques and the introduction of RF ablation catheters with large (4 mm) distal electrode tips, the success rate of this technique improved significantly compared to that reported in initial experience. Currently, the use of RF current catheter ablation has increased dramatically in patients with supraventricular tachycardia, including AV nodal reentrant tachycardia and AV reciprocating tachycardia with or without preexcitation, as well as in new subsets of patients such as those with atrial flutter, ectopic atrial tachycardia and ventricular tachycardia.

Mechanisms of RF energy-Induced Myocardial Injury and Effects on Myocardial Tissue

The mechanism of myocardial injury in response to RF current delivery is presumed to be thermal. In addition, it has been suggested that the oscillating electromotive force may exert a direct effect on the myocyte sarcolemmal membrane. Thermal coagulation of about 250 mm^3 of the target tissue occurs in response to electrode-tissue interface temperatures of about 50°C or more;

when temperatures at the electrode-tissue interface reach or exceed 100°C the plasma boils at the electrode surface and an insulating film of coagulated plasma and desiccated tissue forms on the conductive surface. Reduction of effective electrode surface area leads to increased current density, more tissue heating, more coagulum formation and eventual "breakdown" of delivered energy. In clinical practice, early recognition of this phenomenon is made possible by impedance monitoring; if a sudden increase of impedance is observed during pulse delivery, immediate pulse discontinuation is mandatory to reduce the risk of thrombus formation. Anticoagulation with intravenous heparin is also performed in most centers to minimize the risk of thrombus formation and its complications.

Four to five days after ablation the center of the lesion shows complete coagulation necrosis and early fatty changes, whereas a discrete border between living and dead tissue replaces the inflammatory transition zone observed acutely. It is likely that changes occurring in the transition zone are, at least in part, responsible for late success or late recurrence, depending on the evolution during this phase. By 8 weeks, the chronic lesion has been replaced by fibrosis and shows evidence of contraction and marked volume loss. The border zone of the lesion is well defined without any patchy necrosis or islands of viable myocardium. The uniform nature and the small volume of the lesion likely account for the low rate of reported late arrhythmic and non-arrhythmic complications from RF current catheter ablation.

Efficacy of RF Current Ablation in Patients with Accessory Pathways

Currently success rates well exceeding 90% are being reported by experienced centers for RF current ablation of supraventricular tachycardias secondary to an accessory atrioventricular pathway. Two prerequisites must be fulfilled to make this strategy successful. First, precise localization of the accessory pathway. Recently developed catheter techniques allow, if properly searched for, direct recording of accessory pathway activation from the distal electrode pair at the tip of the mapping/ablation catheter [17]. Radiofrequency current delivery to sites of accessory pathway activation potential recording, especially if associated with other local electrogram parameters suggestive of early local activation [18], almost always results in immediate conduction block within the accessory pathway. Often, very few RF current pulses are required to produce accessory pathway interruption. This underlines the importance of precise mapping techniques, as compared to the surgical approach [1] where extended areas along the atrioventricular annuli are frequently excised to minimize recurrence.

Second, the introduction of specially designed catheters with a steerable tip that can be freely manoeuvered from the outside has allowed easier and more precise positioning at any site along the atrioventricular annuli. The large-tip electrode of these catheters also allows delivery of higher energies to the myocardial tissue, thus resulting in a significantly higher success rate than that reported with small (2 mm) distal electrode tips [12].

Catheter maneouvering under fluoroscopic guidance also has important implications for optimizing catheter-tissue contact and stability over time during RF current pulses; this is a crucial issue to maximize the probability of success [19-21]. Several techniques have been proposed to optimize catheter-tissue contact at the atrioventricular annuli. For left-sided accessory pathways either the transaortic retrograde or the transseptal approach can be safely used with similar reported efficacy [22]; in principle, they aim at interrupting accessory pathway conduction at the ventricular and atrial insertion sites, respectively. Right-sided accessory pathways can at times present a challenge to the interventional electrophysiologist. A long-term success rate for RF current catheter ablation in this set of pathways also exceeds 90%, but multiple sessions may be required because of a lower success rate during the first procedure and a relatively high recurrence rate.

Anatomical differences of the tricuspid as opposed to the mitral annulus likely account for the difficulties encountered while attempting RF current ablation of right-sided accessory pathways; they include a larger mappable circumference (ca. 12 cm of the tricuspid annulus versus ca. 10 cm of the mitral annulus in the normal adult), an annular development less pronounced with discontinuities of the fibrous skeleton, a more acute angle between the endocardium and the valve leaflet, the presence of Ebstein's anomaly or of Mahaim-like fibers accounting for about 10% of all right-sided accessory pathways, and, most importantly, the absence along the annulus of a conveniently accessible venous structure for mapping. In selected cases, the right coronary artery may be used to advance properly designed catheter electrodes and map along the epicardial right atrioventricular groove in search of the accessory pathway location.

Once the accessory pathway has been localized several techniques may be used to maximize catheter-tissue contact and stability depending on the target site along the tricuspid annulus. In our center anteroseptal, anterior and anterolateral accessory pathways are most easily accessed using an approach from the superior vena cava (entrance either from the internal jugular vein or right subclavian vein); accessory pathways in the right lateral, posterolateral, posterior, posteroseptal and midseptal positions are initially approached using a catheter inserted through the right femoral vein and into the inferior vena cava. Additional techniques can be used in selected cases, including the support of a long sheath embedding the mapping catheter from the entry site to the inferior vena cava ostium and a looping technique allowing the catheter tip to approach the accessory pathway from the subannular site.

After successful ablation of an accessory pathway, careful monitoring is required before discharge to control the patient's clinical condition and exclude pericardial reaction. Recurrence is observed in about 5% of patients during follow-up; repeated procedures are generally recommended in such cases and result in definitive abolition of the accessory pathway.

Complications of RF Current Ablation Techniques

General Complications

The complication rate of RF catheter ablation procedures is about 5%; it includes complications related to catheter manipulation and to RF current delivery. Among complications are inadvertent complete atrioventricular nodal block, pericardial effusion, cardiac tamponade, coronary artery spasm or thrombosis, intracavitary thrombus formation, thromboembolism, pneumothorax, aortic wall dissection, local hemathoma, and arterovenous fistulae. In cooperative reports, the incidence of complications was 3.8% in a large American collective [23] and 4.4% in the European MERFS survey [24]. In the latter study life-threatening complications such as tamponade and embolism were reported in 0.7% and 0.6% of cases respectively. A procedure-related death has occasionally been reported in patients undergoing RF current ablation.

Complications Related to the Location of the Accessory Pathway

Inadvertent complete atrioventricular nodal block has been reported in patients undergoing ablation of accessory pathways located in the septal space. Some precautions can be taken to minimize this risk whenever RF current last to be delivered in the midseptal or anteroseptal region; they include 1) selection of the venous access associated with the greatest catheter stability at these sites, 2) use of a temperature-controlled mode with initial pre-set values not exceeding 55-60°C, 3) careful monitoring of atrial retrograde conduction if junctional ectopic rhythm ensues during RF current applications, with immediate discontinuation of pulse delivery in case of a retrograde (ventriculoatrial) block, and 4) early discontinuation of energy delivery for pulses which fail to produce an early accessory pathway conduction block.

Accessory pathways ablated from within the coronary sinus or its tributary veins are referred to as epicardial accessory pathways; they account for about 5% of all left-sided accessory pathways. Radiofrequency current pulses delivered inside the cardiac venous system should be titrated at low power (not exceeding 15 Watts/sec) or low pre-set temperature (not exceeding 55-60°C). In case of a sudden impedance rise during pulse delivery, which may not infrequently be observed due to a less pronounced cooling effect by the circulating blood in this region, immediate pulse discontinuation is mandatory to minimize the risk of thrombus formation and catheter adhesion to the venous wall. Despite these safety measures, thrombosis may nevertheless develop leading occasionally to occlusion of the coronary sinus; in our experience, this event has never been associated with clinical complications and complete recanalization could be documented a few days after the procedure. Thus far, there are no reports of perforation produced by RF current delivered within the cardiac veins leading to pericardial effusion or tamponade.

Potential Hazards of RF Current Catheter Ablation

A potential source of risk to the patient and the investigators performing RF current catheter ablation procedures is the radiation exposure from fluoroscopic imaging required to guide catheter manipulation. The estimated absorbed dose per RF ablation procedure in a high volume American center was 2.5 rem in the breast, 2.0 rem in the active bone marrow and 7.5 rem in the lungs [25]. These figures would lead to a lifetime risk of excess malignancies per 1 million patients undergoing 60 minutes fluoroscopy of 150 (females only), 120 and 710 respectively (a 0.07% lifetime risk of developing a fatal malignancy due to radiation exposure). In addition, the risk estimation for autosomal dominant abnormalities in the first generation is 5 to 35 cases per 1 million liveborn per absorbed rem, and the risk for all genetic disorders less than 50 cases per million liveborn per absorbed rem. Although difficult to translate to clinical practice, these estimates outline the necessity of minimizing fluoroscopy time during RF current catheter ablation procedures without reducing efficacy and safety. The volume of exposed body weight and the life expectancy with respect to the effective clinical benefit should also be taken into account at the time of patient selection.

In patients in whom RF current delivery in the proximity of the atrioventricular node is performed to ablate an accessory pathway, long term follow-up is recommended to evaluate the potential impact of fibrotic lesions on atrioventricular conduction.

Indications for RF Current Catheter Ablation of Accessory Pathways

Radiofrequency is currently the energy source of choice for ablation of accessory atrioventricular pathways. It is highly effective and carries a low risk. Owing to these properties, it has been proposed as a therapy for patients with incessant or drug-refractory tachycardias mediated by an accessory pathway and for symptomatic patients who refuse lifelong drug therapy [23]. In asymptomatic patients with Wolff-Parkinson-White syndrome, the decision to ablate the accessory pathway should be an individual one, based on electrophysiological data, type of occupation or physical activities of the patient, and the patient's personal motivation. In children, the benefits of this therapy should be carefully counterbalanced with the risks related to complications and fluoroscopy exposure, as well as by taking into account the not infrequent disappearance of the accessory pathway during growth [26]; at our center patients of age younger than 4 years or with a body weight lower than 50 kg are candidates to accessory pathway ablation only in cases of incessant or drug refractory tachycardias in the presence of left ventricular dysfunction.

RF Current Catheter Ablation as the Therapy of Choice in Patients with Reciprocating Atrioventricular Tachycardia?

It has been estimated that the risk of sudden death in asymptomatic patients with Wolff-Parkinson-White syndrome is about 0.1% per patient-year [27]; this figure may increase to 0.56% per patient-year in patients with an accessory pathway capable of rapid conduction during atrial fibrillation. Sudden death may be the first manifestation of Wolff-Parkinson-White syndrome in 25% of cases [28]. In addition, in about 10% of sudden arrhythmic deaths in young people with an apparently normal heart who have never undergone a clinical investigation, histologic examination may disclose an anatomical alteration consistent with preexcitation [29]. An electrophysiologic investigation helps to identify those patients at low risk of ventricular fibrillation and should be performed routinely in patients with Wolff-Parkinson-White syndrome; this procedure carries an inherent risk of complication and in experienced centers the possibility of concomitant cure by means of RF current ablation is offered to the patient during the same session. Transesophageal electrophysiologic study is used as a surrogate of the intracavitary diagnostic procedure in some centers.

Antiarrhythmic drug therapy has long been used in the chronic treatment of patients with reciprocating atrioventricular tachycardia. The clinical efficacy of these agents in highly symptomatic patients ranges between 70% and 100%, although only about 50% of them become asymptomatic [30]. In addition, antiarrhythmic drug therapy is associated with a 3% to 34% risk of proarrhythmia which at times may be fatal [31-34]. Also, the use of these drugs does not necessarily prevent patients with Wolff-Parkinson-White syndrome from sudden death [28]. Additional organ toxicity is seen with all antiarrhythmic agents and has an incidence as high as 26% in the case of amiodarone [35]. Not infrequently, patients with Wolff-Parkinson-White syndrome or reciprocating atrioventricular tachycardias are women of childbearing age; in such cases, the risk of congenital defects resulting from pregnancy occurring in the presence of an antiarrhythmic agent must also be taken into account.

Sudden Cardiac Death in Athletes and its Relationship to WPW Syndrome

The concept that highly trained athletes may die suddenly of cardiac causes is somewhat a paradox, as this group represents the population in which cardiovascular performance and fitness are supposed to be optimal. It is probably for this reason and because athletes have become rather reference symbols in most societies that sudden death even in a small number of athletes receives great public attention. Among the dominant factors underlying sudden cardiac death in athletes are hypertrophic cardiomyopathy and coronary artery disease (both congenital and acquired); among other causes, WPW syndrome, long QT syndrome and mitral valve prolapse or aortic rupture may lead to sudden cardiac death.

In the athlete with WPW syndrome, the risk of sudden death during strenuous effort may relate to the shortening of the accessory pathway anterograde refractoriness secondary to enhanced plasma levels of sympathetic hormones. Though objective evidence is lacking, the sequence of events leading to sudden death during effort in athletes with WPW syndrome is probably as follows: onset of atrial fibrillation (spontaneous or secondary to degeneration from a reciprocating atrioventricular tachycardia) with fast anterograde conduction through the accessory pathway with high ventricular rate with asymmetric depolarization and repolarization (wide QRS complex on the surface ECG) with degeneration into ventricular fibrillation.

In athletes, the risk of sudden death is more difficult to assess compared to that of the general WPW syndrome patient population. Among the causes for this are the inability to reproduce the autonomic and hormonal changes which occur during maximal effort in the EP laboratory; the inability of provocative tests such as intravenous isoproterenol or atropine to trigger life-threatening arrhythmias in the EP laboratory does not exclude the risk of sudden death secondary to ventricular fibrillation in the clinical setting.

Conclusions

From these data it is evident that RF current catheter ablation is an optimal tool to cure patients with an accessory pathway. Among individuals with Wolff-Parkinson-White syndrome, identification of those at risk of developing ventricular fibrillation is mandatory and should be undertaken by means of an electrophysiologic study; at this time ablation of any accessory pathway is, in experienced hands, easily feasible in more than 90% of cases and should be offered to the patient as an option provided that he/she has been correctly informed about the pathophysiology and the risk of his/her disease, as well as the risks of the therapeutic procedure.

In athletes, the advantages of radiofrequency ablation are remarkable in so far that this technique cures the anatomic and electrophysiologic substrate responsible for generation of supraventricular into ventricular arrhythmias; this in turn allows the athlete to retourn to full activity without risk of sudden cardiac death.

References

1. Cobb RF, Blumenschein SD, Sealy WC et al (1968) Successful surgical interruption of the bundle of Kent in a patient with Wolff-Parkinson-White syndrome. Circulation 38: 1018-1029
2. Scheinman MM, Morady F, Hess DS et al (1982) Catheter-induced ablation of the atrioventricular junction to control refractory supraventricular arrhythmias. JAMA 248: 851-855
3. Haissaguerre M, Warin JF, Lemetayer P et al (1989) Closed-chest ablation of retro-

grade conduction in patients with atrioventricular nodal reentrant tachycardia. N Engl J Med 320: 851-855

4. Brugada P, de Swart H, Smeets JL, Wellens HJ (1989) Transcoronary chemical ablation of ventricular tachycardia. Circulation 79: 475-482

5. Littman L, Svenson RH, Tomcsanyi et al (1991) Modification of atrioventricular nodal transnission properties by intraoperative neodymium-YAG laser photocoagulation in dogs. J Am Coll Cardiol 17: 797-804

6. Gillette PC, Swindle MM, Thompson RF, Case CL (1991) Transvenous cryoablation of the bundle of His. PACE 14: 504-510

7. Haines DE, Whayne JG (1992) What is the radial temperature profile achieved during microwave catheter ablation with a helical coil antenna in canine myocardium? J Am Coll Cardiol 19:99A

8. He D, Zimmer JE, Hynynen KH et al (1992) Application of ultrasound energy tfor intracardiac ablation of arrhythmias. Circulation 86 I-783

9. Borggrefe M, Buddle T, Podzeck A, Breithardt (1987) High frequency alternatin current ablation of an acessory pathway in humans. J Am Coll Cardiol 10:576-582

10. Kuck KH, Kunze KP, Schlüter M, Geiger M, Jackman WM, Naccarelli GV (1988) Modification of a left-sided accessory atrioventricular pathway by raiofrequency current using a bipolar epicardial-endocardial electrode configuration. Eur Heart J 9:927-932

11. Jackman WM, Wang X, Friday KJ, Roman CA, Moulton KP, Beckman KJ, McClelland JH, Twidale N, Hazlitt A, Prior MI, Margolis PD, Calame JD, Overholt ED, Lazzara R (1991) Catheter ablation of accessory atrioventricular pathways (Wolff-Parkinson-White syndrome) by radiofrequency current. N Engl J Med 324:1605-1611

12. Kuck KH, Schlüter M, Geiger M, Siebels J, Duckeck W (1991) Radiofrequency current catheter ablation of accessory atrioventricular pathways. Lancet 337:1557-1561

13. Calkins H, Sousa J, Rosenheck S, de Buitleir M, Kou WH, Kadish AH, Langberg JJ, Morady F (1991) Diagnosis and cure of the Wolff-Parkinson-White syndrome or paroxysmal supraventricular tachycardias during a single electrophysiologic test. N Engl J Med 324:1612-1618

14. Schlüter M, Geiger M, Siebels J, Duckeck W, Kuck KH (1991) Catheter ablation using radiofrequency current to cure symptomatic patients with tachyarrhythmias related to an accessory atrioventricular pathway. Circulation 84:1644-1661

15. Leather RA, Leitch JW, Klein GJ, Guiraudon GM, Yee R, Kim YH (1991) Radiofrequency catheter ablation of accessory pathways: a learning experience. Am J Cardiol 68:1651-1655

16. Lesh MD, Van Hare GF, Schamp DJ, Chien W, Lee MA, Griffin JC, Langberg JJ, Cohen TJ, Lurie KG, Scheinman MM (1992) Curative percutaneous catheter ablation using radiofrequency energy for accessory pathways in all locations: results in 100 consecutive patients. J Am Coll Cardiol 19:1303-1309

17. Jackman WM, Friday KJ, Yeung-Lai-Wah JA, Fitzgerald DM, Beck B, Bowman AJ, Stelzer P, Harrison L, Lazzara R (1988) New catheter technique for recording left free-wall accessory atrioventricular pathway activation. Identification of pathway fiber orientation. Circulation 78:598-610

18. Cappato R, Schlüter M, Mont L, Kuck KH (1994) Anatomic, electrical, and mechanical factors affecting bipolar endocardial electrograms: impact on catheter ablation of manifest left free-wall accessory pathways. Circulation 90:884-894

19. Calkins H, Kim YN, Schmaltz S, Sousa J, el-Atassi R, Leon A, Kadish A, Langberg JJ, Morady F (1992) Electrogram criteria for identification of appropriate target sites for radiofrequency catheter ablation of accessory atrioventricular connections.

Circulation 85:565-573
20. Chen X, Borggrefe M, Shenasa M, Haverkamp W, Hindricks G, Breithardt G (1992) Characteristics of local electrogram predicting successful transcatheter radiofrequency ablation of left-sided accessory pathways. J Am Coll Cardiol 20:656-665
21. Silka MJ, Kron J, Halperin BD, Griffith K, Crandall B, Oliver RP, Walance CG, McAnulty JH (1992) Analysis of local electrogram characteristics correlated with successful radiofrequency catheter ablation of accessory atrioventricular pathways. PACE Pacing Clin Electrophysiol 15:1000-1007
22. Ma C, Dong J, Yang X, Shang L, Iiu X, Sun Y, Hu D (1995) A randomized comparison between retrograde and transseptal approach for radiofrequency ablation of left-sided accessory pathways. PACE 18:915II
23. Scheinman MM (1992) Catheter ablation for cardiac arrhythmias, personnel and facilities. PACE 15:715-721
24. Hindricks G (1993) The multicentre European radiofrequency survey. Complications of radiofrequency catheter ablation of arrhythmias. Eur Heart J 14:256-262
25. Calkins H, Niklason L, Sousa J, El-Atassi R, Langberg J, Morady F (1991) Radiation exposure during radiofrequency ablation of accessory atrioventricrualr connections. Circulation 84:2376-2382
26. Perry JC, Garson A (1990) Supraventricular tachycardia de to the Wolff-Parkinson-White syndrome in children: early disappearance and late recurrence. J Am Coll Cardiòl 16:1215-1220
27. Klein GJ, Prystowski EN, Sharma AD, Laupacis A (1989) Asymptomatic Wolff-Parkinson-White syndrome: should we intervene? Circulation 80:1902-1905
28. Torner Montoya P, Brugada P Smeets J, Talajic M, Della Bella P, Lezaun R, Dool A, Wellens HJJ, Bayes de Luna A, Oter R, Breitardt G, Borggrefe M, Klein H, Kuck KH, Kunze KP, Coumel P, Leclercq JF, Chouty F, Frank R, Fontaine G (1991) Ventricular fibrillation in the Wolff-Parkinson-White syndrome: Eur Heart J 12:144-150
29. Corrado D, Basso C, Angelini A, Thiene G (1995) Sudden "arrhythmic" death in young people with apparently normal heart. J Am Coll Cardiol 188A
30. Henthorn RW, Waldo AL, Anderson JL, Gilbert EM, Alpert BL, Bhandari AK, Hawkinson AW, Pritchett EL (1991) Flecainide acetate prevents recurrence of symptomatic paroxysmal supraventricular tachycardia. The flecainide supraventricular tachycardia study group. Circulation 83:119-125
31. Creamer JE, Nathan AW, Camm AJ (1987) The proarrhythmic effects of antiarrhythmic drugs. Am Heart J 2:397-406
32. Velebit V, Podrid P, Lown B, Cohen BH. Graboys TB (1982) Aggravation and provocation of ventricular arrhythmias by antiarrhythmic drugs. Circulation 65:886-894
33. Coplen SE, Antman EM, Berlin JA, Hewitt P, Chalmers TC (1990) Efficacy and safety of quinidine therapy for manteinance of sinus rhythm after cardioversio: A meta-analysis of randomized control trials. Circulation 82:1106-1116
34. The Cardiac Arrhythmia Suppression Trial (CAST) Investigators (1989) Preliminary report. Effect encainide and flecainide on mortality in a randomized trial of arrhythmia suppression after myocardial infarction. N Engl J Med 321:406-412
35. Mason JW (1987) Amiodarone. N Engl J Med 316:455-466

The Long QT Syndrome

R. Cappato

II Medical Department, St. Georg Hospital, Hamburg, Germany

Congenital and acquired long QT syndromes (CLQTS's) have similar features and *torsade de pointes* is the arrhythmia they have in common. Such arrhythmia, generally self-limiting, can sometimes result in ventricular fibrillation and cause sudden death.

Since 1975 [1], the term congenital long QT syndrome has been used to indicate two different forms: one associated with deafness (Jerwell and Lange-Nielsen's syndrome) and characterized by a recessive transmission trait, the other one, a sporadic form, is not associated with deafness (Romano-Ward syndrome) and has a dominant transmission trait.

The overall clinical and scientific interest in the long QT syndrome is due to the peculiarities of the disease, that is: 1) the seriousness of the clinical picture, characterized by syncope, generally taking place during the performance of hard physical exercise and often resulting in a cardiac arrest or in the sudden death of young and apparently healthy subjects; 2) it gives the possibility to study a peculiar physiopathologic model of non-coronaric neural sudden death; 3) it is generally believed that a full understanding of the long QT syndrome's physiopathology can give a major contribution to the comprehension of the mechanisms employed by the neurovegetative system to foster or prevent the onset of malignant ventricular arrhythmia.

In addition to the QT interval's prolongation, the most common electrocardiographic changes characterizing the long QT syndrome are: increase of QT interval's dispersion [3, 4], lower heart rate than healthy subjects of the same age and gender [5, 6], presence of sinus pauses (generally not preceded by changes in the sinus rate) and the T wave alternation, that is an intermittent change (every second beat) of its polarity, often preceding the onset of the *torsade de pointes* [7].

Physiopathogenesis

The Hypothesis of the Sympathetic Imbalance

According to this theory, the neurovegetative tone of the right sympathic axis is lower than normal due to hyper-activity of the left axis' sympathic nerves. In laboratory, it is possible to reproduce an imbalance between the two nervous sections, as well as a significant similitude with the electrocardiographic symptoms of the long QT syndrome, removing the right stellate ganglion or stimulating the left stellate ganglion.

The Hypothesis of the Endocardiac Anomaly

The theory of the endocardiac anomaly is based on the fact that the QT interval's changes and the ventricular arrhythmias which characterize the congenital long QT syndrome are similar to those shown by some acquired forms, as a consequence of the reduction of the K^+ transmembrane conduction (as side effect of class III antiarrhythmic drugs or cesius, or as in cases of a reduction in calcium activity - hypocalcemia - or in the extracellular potassium activity - hypopotassemia). This reduction can result both in a facilitation of the triggered activity, able to produce a repetitive ectopic beats, and in the creation of conditions enhancing a functional re-entry; both these mechanisms could independently result in the ventricular arrhythmias of long QT syndrome affected patients.

It is important to underline that the theory described first (the theory of the sympathetic imbalance) doesn't exclude the theory of an anomaly of the conduction to the transmembrane ionic currents; it is highly probable that the neurovegetative imbalance can affect the metabolic-electric homeostasis of the cardiac cell. On the contrary, the transmembrane conduction anomaly alone can't explain many issues linked to experimental and clinical results obtained on sympathetic ganglia.

Epidemiology

Incidence

LQTS's incidence is not well known. The congenital form associated with deafness affects 2‰ - 3‰ of born deaf people. Its prevalence is 6% - 10%, but it is possible that its real prevalence is underestimated, due to the fact that this malignant disease can result in sudden death even before it is detected.

The age of the first syncope is lower in males (about 11 years vs. about 16 years); sex distribution is similar until the age of 15, then females are more affected [8].

Clinics

Long QT syndrome can result in syncope or cardiac arrest; victims of the disease are generally young subjects experiencing emotional stress or physical exercise; these patients' surface ECG allows the detection of a prolonged QT interval. Without treatment, these subjects can be victims of syncope relapses, which in most cases cause the patients' death.

In kindred patients affected with long QT syndrome, it is often possible to detect the peculiar electrocardiographic anomaly, as well as a positive case history for syncope or sudden death during youth. The triggering of such symptoms during physical exercise or experience of an emotional stress is a rule. The presence of such symptoms determines the diagnosis of the disease.

Prognosis

Death incidence in patients affected with non-treated long QT syndrome is 5% during each year of the 5 years' follow-up [1]. In subjects victims of at least one syncope episode, mortality is 20% one year after the symptom, over 50% after 15 years [8]. These data are even more impressive if one considers that the first syncope episode generally takes place when the subject is about 14. Treatment of these patients with beta-blocker therapy and/or left stellectomy has deeply changed these patients' prognosis as shown by the fact that long-term mortality is less than 1% each year.

Diagnosis

Long QT syndrome's diagnostic criteria have been summarized in Table 1. LQTS' s diagnosis is made in presence of two major criteria or one major and two minor criteria.

Table 1. LQTS's diagnostic criteria

Major criteria	Minor criteria
Prolonged QT interval (QTc>440msec)	Congenital deafness
	Episodes of electrical alternation
Stress-induces syncope	Low heart rate (in children)
Family members with long QT	Abnormal ventricular repolarization

Therapy

Apart from the primary anomaly responsible for the long QT syndrome's pathogenesis, most episodes are triggered by a sudden sympathic hyper-tone, mainly supported by the left cardiac nerves. The treatment with antiadrenergic agents is the most efficient one in the prevention of the symptoms and in the enhancement of these subjects' prognosis.

The beta-blocker therapy has shown its efficacy reducing distance mortality from 71 % to 6% [9]. Nevertheless, this therapy is not able to control the symptoms and to enhance the prognosis in 20% cases. In such situations, the left stellectomy is recommended and its clinical efficacy has been proved; we can suggest the hypothesis that an adrenergic alpha blocker mechanism is responsible for the onset of the LQTS's ventricular arrhythmias [10]. It should be noted that in men the left stellectomy can be done without the need to ablate the cephalic portion of the left stellate ganglion; in this way it is possibile to avoid the syndrome of Horner.

In a minority of cases syncope takes place during sleep and arrhythmia is pause-dipendent; in such cases a pacemaker can be used together with a pharmacologic and/or surgical therapy.

The use of the implanted automatic defibrillator is recommended only in some particular cases; pharmacologic therapy and/or surgery's efficiency as well as the brief spontaneous length of *torsade de pointes* arrhythmias make it useless if not even dangerous to treat these subjects with such therapy.

References

1. Schwartz PJ, Periti M, Malliani A (1975) The long QT syndrome. Am Heart J 89:378
2. Crampton RS, Schwartz PJ (1978) Some aspects of sudden cardiac death. In: Schwartz PJ, Brown AM, Malliani A Zanchetti A (eds) Neural mechanisms in Cardiac Arrhythmias. New York, Raven Press, pp 1-6
3. Priori SG, Napolitano C, Diehl L, Schwartz PJ (1994) Dispersion of the QT interval. A marker of therapeutic efficacy in the idiopathic long QT syndrome. Circulation 89:1681
4. Day CP, Comb JM, Campbell RWF (1990) QT dispersion: an indication of arrhythmia risk in patients with long QT intervals. Br Heart J 63:342
5. Vincent GM (1986) The heart rate of Romano-Ward syndrome patients. Am Heart J 112:61
6. Locati E, Pancaldi A, Pala M, et al (1988) Exercise-induced electrocardiographic changes in patients with long QT syndrome. Circulation 78 (II):42
7. Schwartz PJ, Malliani A (1975) Electrical alternation of the T wave: Clinical and experimental evidence of its relationship with the sympathetic nervous system and with the long QT syndrome. Am Heart J 89:45
8. Locati EH, Moss AJ, Schwartz PJ et al (1992) Age and gender differences in congenital long QT syndrome: A study in 328 LQTS families. J Am Coll Cardiol 19:367 A
9. Schwartz PJ, Locati E (1985) The idiopathic long QT syndrome. Pathogenetic mechanisms and therapy. Eur Heart J 6 (D):103
10. Schwartz PJ (1985) Idiopathic long QT syndrome: Progress and question. Am Heart J 109:309-319

Current Criteria for Evaluation of Athletes with Arrhythmias

F. Furlanello, A. Bertoldi[1], F. Fernando[2]

San Raffaele Scientific Institute, Milan, Italy
[1]Division of Cardiology, S. Chiara Hospital, Trento, Italy
[2]Sport Sciences Institute, Italian National Olympic Committee, Rome, Italy

Cardiac arrhythmias represent a very important and complicated clinical condition especially when one has to consider the eligibility of a subject to take part in competitive sport activities [1, 2]. This is so for a series of reasons:
1. Arrhythmias represent 25-35% of the cardiovascular causes of non eligibility of an athlete after 1st level evaluation and therefore request further investigations (1st level evaluation is that requested annually by Italian law for anyone to take part in competitive sport activities. It involves family and personal history, cardiological evaluation, resting ECG, step test, urine test, spirometry).
2. They are the cause of important sports related symptoms of varying severity.
a) Not potentially dangerous but sufficient to disturb athletic performance and at times the athlete's sports career, due to excessive bradycardia or tachycardia especially if sudden, long lasting and recurrent. Examples are abrupt and long lasting rhythmic or arrhythmic cardiopalmus due to re-entrant supraventricular tachyarrhythmia, junctional or atrial or atrio ventricular (due to manifest or concealed WPW), cathecolamine or vagal induced atrial fibrillation, sinus bradyarrhythmias (SA) or recovery AV, "incessant" supraventricular and ventricular tachyarrhythmias, prolonged bigeminism usually present at medium and low intensity exercise.
b) Life threatening tachyarrhythmias such as to induce fainting, vertigo, syncope and cardiac arrest (CA) which if not resuscitated can lead to sudden death [2-7]. Examples include torsade de pointe (TdP), rapid sustained ventricular polymorphic or haemodynamically unstable VT, rapid preexcited AF in WPW and VF that usually represents the final stage of malignant hyperkinetic arrhythmias. Also SA and AV asystole (even due to violent reflex stimuli such as concussio cordis, or severe cardioinhibitory neuro-reflex syndrome) [14].
3. Arrhythmias can be markers and/or consequences of an underlying arrhythmogenic cardiopathy, which is by itself sufficient to consider the athlete non eligible. The problem is a complex one when the potentially arrhythmogenic cardiopathy is asymptomatic and therefore not easily diagnosed. This is the case in hypertrophic cardiomyopathy (HCM), dilated cardiomyopathy (DCM), arrhythmogenic right ventricular dysplasia (ARVD), congenital or atherosclerotic ischaemic heart disease (IHD), complicated mitral valve prolapse (MVP), certain post surgical arrhythmogenic cardiopathies, myocarditis in its various forms (acute, healing, healed), the primary arrhythmogenic pathologies of the conduction system and those of WPW type, some primary hyperkinetic ma-

lignant ventricular tachyarrhythmias etc. It is possible however that the diagnosed or suspected arrhythmias are independent and coexist with the cardiopathy and therefore have bystander significance. Example are WPW and ventricular ectopic beats, WPW and MVP, MVP and idiopathic right ventricular ectopic beats and functional AV block and ARVD.

4. Cardiac arrhythmias especially the hypokinetic forms "paraphysiologically" induced by systematic athletic activity can modify the physiological atrial, SA and AV terrain and lead in time, if the subject practises sports activity regular intense, to real atrial disease with pathologic AV block and also prepare for the onset of paroxysmal and/or chronic atrial fibrillation in the "older" athlete.

5. The correct classification of cardiac arrhythmias in athletes is not always easy. This is the case both for "benign" or "paraphysiologic" arrhythmias, which can be compatible with sports eligibility, and "pathological" ones which would exclude the patient from sports. The latter must be considered such because of their direct consequences on the athletes performace, the risks, the severe symptoms and/or the fact that they may be markers of an underlying cardiopathy. In addition, morphologically similar arrhythmias can have totally different prognostic significance based on a series of conditions, for example:

a) whether they are in relation with an underlying cardiopathy, for example, VEB's with right bundle branch morphology originating from the right ventricular outflow tract can be idiopathic and benign or an expression of an arrhythmogenic right ventricular dysplasia/cardiomyopathy;

b) atrial fibrillation can be compatible with daily life but incompatible in subjects engaged in sport activity;

c) some arrhythmias can disturb athletic performance even if they are intrinsically benign, for example, high frequency repetitive ventricular tachycardia and posterior left fascicular ventricular tachycardia verapamil like;

d) arrhythmias present in athletes that are engaged in potentially dangerous sport activities, such as re-entrant supraventricular tachyarrhythmias including WPW syndrome in downhill skiing, motor sports, mountain climbing, underwater sports etc.

In conclusion, the evaluation of cardiac arrhythmias in athletes can be summarized:

a. research for an underlying cardiomyopathy, even if only in the initial stage, which could be potentially arrhythmogenic and "responsible" for the observed arrhythmia;

b. a rational evaluation of the clinical and haemodynamic consequences of the arrhythmia in relation to the athlete's career.

These problems are in many cases far from easy even when the patients are referred to expert Centres, particularly as regards the research of an underlying arrhythmogenic cardiopathy in its initial phase but potentially severe and/or progressive. In addition, there are arrhythmic situations that cannot be classified with certainty, this can lead to an over or underestimation of the prognosis, for example in borderline forms of WPW or complex hyperkinetic ventricular arrhythmias, especially if the VEB's are numerous and accompanied by episodes of non sustained VT. The COCIS '95 [8] and the Bethesda Conference '94 [9] dealt with the problem of cardiac arrhythmias from different points of view. COCIS '95 gave direct responsability to the sports physicians in relation to sport eligibility, while the Bethesda Conference '94 self-responsibilizes the athlete following advice based on clinical and cardiological experience. COCIS '95, both for cardiac arrhythmias and the other cardiovascular situations covered, sets out a cardiological "guideline" in relation to the decision for sports eligibility. With respect to the 1989 version it introduces some new aspects concerning cardiac arrhythmias, due to the progress achieved in sports arrhythmology and also from the suggestions and requests from sports physicians [2, 10, 11] of particular interest:

1.) A more detailed classification of the three levels of cardioarrhythmological evaluation aimed at assessing athlete's eligibility. This is useful to define specific tasks and establish guidelines for the diagnostic evaluation of the arrhythmic athlete. The cardioarrhytmologic protocol of the athlete includes:

- *1st level evaluation.* Performed during the first visit that an athlete must undergo and includes family history, clinical examination with ECG and stress test (step test). Following this evaluation 3-4% of the athletes are usually considered non eligible of which 60-80% due to cardiovascular reasons and of these 25-35% for arrhythmic causes.

- *2 nd level evaluation.* Consists of an echocardiographic study, possibly with Doppler colour flow, maximal stress test and 24 hour ECG recording. The latter must also include a period of intense physical activity (preferably the athletes specific sport activity) so as to achieve maximum heart rate. Usually one also performs thyroid function evaluation (T3, T4, FT4 and TSH), blood electrolytes (sodium and potassium) and if there is suspicion of an underlying infectious disease one will also carry out tests for rheumatic activity and viral infections.

- *3rd level evaluation.* This level includes specific invasive and non invasive cardioarrhythmologic investigations carried out depending on the type of documented or suspected arrhythmia. There is also a re-evaluation of the 2nd level results through examinations which include ventricular late potentials (VLP), both in time and frequency domain (if possible), and a tilt test. They also include transesophageal atrial pacing (TAP) at rest and during exercise for inducible supraventricular tachyarrhythmias, such as re-entrant tachycardia, atrial fibrillation, WPW and as an initial screening for hypokinetic arrhythmias (SA and AV). Finally there is an endocavitary electrophysiologic study, used as a method to evaluate the conduction system in athletes with hypokinetic SA and pre-and post-Hissian AV arrhythmias, and for the research of atrial and ventricular irritability even utilising aggressive protocols.
In addition a series of non invasive and invasive diagnostic techniques are performed in athletes with arrhythmias to rule out the presence of an under-

lying cardiac disease; in particular tests for an arrhytmogenic substate. These tests for underlying cardiopathy can also include stress and transesophageal echocardiography, nuclear scintigraphy at rest and during exercise, 123 MIBG SPECT, NMR, cardiac catheterisation and coronarography and myocardial biopsy. In addition the possible research for underlying infectious diseases with particular focus on viral causes and specific tests to detect the intake of arrhythmogenic substances.

From our cardioarrhythmologic study of 132 top level athletes between 1985-1995, 109 males and 23 females of average age 23.6, who underwent 3rd level cardioarrhytmological evaluation for important manifest or documented arrhytmic manifestations, 71/132 (53.7%) were considered eligible to take part in competitive sports activities and 61/132 (46.3%) were considered non eligible. Of these, 14 (22.9%), were placed on antiarrhythmic treatment due to the severity of the arrhythmia and/or the underlying cardiopathy. A World Champion cyclist died suddenly during sports activity 3 yrs. after having undergone a cardioarrhytmologic evaluation and after which is was considered non eligible (Table 1) [12].

Table 1. Results of 132 top level athletes followed-up for 1 -135 months

	N°	%
Eligible to take part in competitive sport activities	71	53.7
Non eligible to take part in competitive sport activities	61	46.3

Of these

14 (22.9%) on AAD treatment (= 10.6% of 132 TLA)

1 had sudden death during sports activity

2.) A means to extend the criteria for eligibility in subjects with arrhythmias especially in the absence of an underlying cardiopathy, therefore giving 3rd level consultation a greater decisional capacity. This owing to the new diagnostic tools and further knowledge of arrhythmias relevant in athletes, for example, congenital AV block or primary idiopathic VT such as iterative VT and fascicular VT.

3.) The acceptance of possibility of recovery even with malignant hyperkinetic arrhythmias including cardiac arrest, in cases where there is an identifiable cause without subsequent sequele such as myocarditis, concussio cordis or WPW after RFC catheter ablation of the anomalous pathway [1, 7].

4.) The particular attention paid to myocarditis, as the existence of a silent pathology, dangerous but also totally resolvable, is frequently encountered in athletes of every age [13].

5.) Special attention should be given to the "appendix" chapter (COCIS '95) concerning electrical therapies as a new diagnostic tool in the evaluation of arrhythmic athletes and their eligibility. In particular a better codification of transcatheter ablation, which at present utilises RF, but in the future will probably use other forms of energy to improve the "recovery" phase of the patient with tachyarrythmias and incorporate the precautions needed to avoid potentially dangerous side effects. It also addresses the possibility of giving eligibility in selected cases, such as patients with PM, in whom the hypokinetic arrhythmia is primary, in the absence of other cardiopathies, and has been corrected for the athletes performance. Also one must remember ICDs (implantable cardioverter defibrillators) utilised in ex-athletes with otherwise intractable malignant hyperkinetic arrhytmias.

The Bethesda Conference 1994 represents an incredible focus on the arrhythmic manifestations that can be met in athletes and that have consequences for the sport activity in the short, medium and long range. However, the absence the American cardiologist's direct responsibility conditions a series of permissive behaviours that would be unacceptable for the Italian cardiolo-gist. However, the ever increasing numbers of cardiac arrests and sudden death in athletes with arrhythmogenic cardiopathies which were apparently insignificant and functionally compatible with even strenuous competitive sports activity must make us wary when we have to decide on an arrhythmic athlete's eligibility in the "absence of an underlying cardiopathy", since at times even with 3rd level examinations it can be very difficult to identify the arrhythmogenic substate.

COCIS '95 represents a responsible means of developing clinical and instrumental "guidelines" (still improvable) for the arrhythmic athlete, in the light of the progress of clinical arrhythmology and sport in order to protect his profession and safeguard him from the sport activity. This keeping in mind, in a critical but open way, the suggestions of our American Colleagues for whom decisional tasks are easier since there are no direct medical legal aspects such as those in Italy.

References

1. Furlanello F, Bertoldi A, Bettini R, Dallago M, Vergara G (1992) Life threatening tachyarrhythmias in athletes. PACE 15:1403-1412
2. Furlanello F, Bertoldi A (1995) Aritmie cardiache ed idoneità agonistica. COCIS 1995 Bethesda Conference 1994. In: Atti VII Congresso Nazionale Società italiana di Cardiologia dello Sport, Trento, 20-2219/1995, Ed. C.E.S.I. pp 41-44
3. Furlanello F, Bettini R, Cozzi F et al (1984) Ventricular arrhythmias and sudden death in athletes. Clinical aspects of life-threatening arrhythmias. Ann N Acad Sci 427:253-279

4. Furlanello F, Bertoldi A, Dallago M, et al (1992) Evaluation of cardiac arrhythmias in athletes. J Ambul Monit 5/4: 2X5-297
5. Furlanello F, Bettini R, Bertoldi A et al (1991) Competitive sports and cardiac arrhythmias. In: B. Lideritz, S. Saksena (eds.); Interventional Electrophysiology. Futura Publishing Inc. Mount Kisco, N.Y., pp 41-47
6. Furlanello F, Bertoldi A, Dallago M, Gramegna L, Vergara G, Befflni R, Inama G (1994) Aborted Sudden Death in Competitive Athletes. Progress in Clinical Pacing 51:733-741
7. Bertoldi A, Furlanello F, Fernando F, Gramegna L, Dallago M, Inama G, Bettini R, Durante GB, Vergara G Young Competitive athletes resuscitated from cardiac arrest on field: what have we learned and what can be done? New Trends Arrhyt. 11 n°1-4:20-30
8. Comitato organizzativo cardiologico per l'idoneita allo sport (COCIS) (1996) Protocolli cardiologici per il giudizio di idoneità allo sport agonistico 1995. G Ital Cardiol, Vol. 26 (in press)
9. 26th Bethesda Conference (1994) Reccomendations for determining eligibility for competition in athletes with cardiovascular abnormalities. J Am Coll Cardiol 24:848-899
10. Furlanello F, Bertoldi A (1996) Protocolli cardiologici per il giudizio di idoneità allo sport agonistico 1995. Introduzione. G Ital Cardiol 26 (in press)
11. Furlanello F, Bertoldi A (1995) Aritmie ventricolari nel sano e nello sportivo agonistico. In: Rovelli F, De Vita C, Moreo A. (eds) Cardiologia. Scientific Press, Firenze: 573-581
12. Bertoldi A, Furlanello F, Fernando F et al (1993) Cardioarrhythmologic evaluation of symptoms and arrhythmic manifestations in 110 top level consecutive professional atheletes. New Trends Arrhyt 9:199-209
13. Zeppilli P (1995) Cardiologia dello Sport. C.E.S.I., Roma
14. Maron BJ, Pollac LC, Kaplan JA, Mueller KO (1993) Blunt impact to the chest leading to sudden death from cardiac arrest during sport activities. N Engl J Med 329:55-57

Congenital Heart Disease of Interest in Athletes

P. Colonna

G. M. Lancisi Hospital, Ancona, Italy

Congenital heart diseases (CHD) relative to sports medicine can be divided into 2 principal groups:
a) "Simple" CHD- generally asymptomatic, in which sports practice is often allowed even before eventual surgical correction.
b) "Complex" CHD- frequently cyanotic and can allow participation in sports only after surgical correction and only in selected cases.

CHD of the first group are more frequent (70%) and can be diagnosed by chance during a medical check for sports practice. To identify the CHD it is important to know their physical manifestations.

CHD of the second group are generally symptomatic and are thus, often diagnosed at neonatal age. The sports physician is involved only with postoperative forms and so should know residual defects and sequele following complex CHD correction.

Congenitally corrected transposition of the great arteries does not fit this scheme as it is an anatomically complex CHD but which, if isolated, may be asymptomatic and of mild haemodynamic significance.

Congenital coronary anomalies are a distinct group of diseases of great importance in sports medicine as they can be related to sudden death.

"Simple" CHD

"Simple" CHD can be subdivided from an haemodynamic point of view into 2 large subgroups:
a) CHD with increased pulmonary blood flow due to a left to right shunt at the-
    atrial level
    ventricular level
    pulmonary level.
b) CHD with obstruction to ventricular outflow-
    pulmonary
    systemic.

CHD with Increased Pulmonary Blood Flow

Atrial Septal Defect

There are various anatomical types:
- the sinus venosus is positioned high in the atrial septum and is frequently associated with partial pulmonary anomalous venous return;
- ostium secundum is the most common and is in an intermediate position;
- the ostium primum is low in position and often associated with the mitral cleft.
    Atrial septal defects (ASD) are most frequently met the CHD in athletes for the following reasons:
- high incidence (10% of all CHD);
- few symptoms, often well tolerated during sports practice;
- mild and shaded physical signs characterised by
        grade I-II/VI ejection systolic murmur at pulmonary area
        II tone widely split and usually fixed
        tricuspid diastolic flow murmur (only if shunt is significant)
    Diagnosis is confirmed by laboratory tests. ECG shows incomplete right bundle branch block, Chest X-ray shows increased pulmonary blood flow and enlargement of the right sections and echocardiography right ventricle and pulmonary artery enlargement, and paradoxical motion of the ventricular septal wall. Direct visualisation of the ASD with 2D-ECHO is also possible, as is demonstration of left to right shunt by color Doppler.

Recommendations

Subjects with small ASD, normal heart chamber dimensions and normal motion of the ventricular septum can practice all competitive sports excluding diving, due to the risk of paradoxical air embolism. Exercise testing and 24 hour ECG monitoring are necessary to exclude associated supraventricular arrhythmias and conduction disturbances.
    Moderate or large defects should be corrected before the subject engages in sports.
    6 months after correction athletes can be allowed to participate in all competitive sports in the verified absence of:
- residual pulmonary hypertension;
- supraventricular arrhythmias and sinus node dysfunction;
- significant dilation of cardiac chambers.
    In the first years after correction one frequently finds a persistence of incomplete right bundle branch block and mild enlargement of the right ventricle with anomalous motion of the ventricular septum that does not indicate residual defects and so does not preclude sports practice.
    The ostium primum type of ASD is a form of atrioventricular septal defect (partial AV canal) and is often associated with mitral regurgitation due to a cleft in the anterior leaflet of the mitral valve.

ECG is a very important diagnostic tool as in all patients it shows a left axis deviation as in other forms of AV canal; incomplete right bundle branch block is also present and in 50% of cases I degree heart block.

Conduction disturbances are also more frequent in postoperative patients than in ASD (*ostium secondum*) and an accurate evaluation with ECHO (for residual mitral regurgitation), 24 hour ambulatory ECG and an exercise tolerance test are necessary before allowing sports practice.

Ventricular Septal Defect

Simple ventricular septal defect (VSD) is the single most common CHD at birth (20%) the natural history depends on the size of the defect. Small defects generally close spontaneously in the first years and also occasionally during adolescence.

Athletes with small VSD are asymptomatic but can easily be detected by the harsh loud holosystolic murmur in the precordial area with a normal second sound. The defect is restrictive and so right ventricular pressure remains normal.

ECG and Chest X-ray are normal and also the heart chamber dimensions; Echo-doppler and Colour echo doppler show a small high velocity flow between the right and left ventricle. If the exercise tolerance test is also normal, practice of all competitive sport can be permitted.

Subjects with medium or large VSD generally present symptoms such as dyspnea, reduced growth and exercise tolerance, frequent respiratory infections and have enlargement of the heart chambers or pulmonary hypertension. They cannot engage in sports and a cardiac catheterization is generally indicated before correction.

Post-operative evaluation (at least 6 months after intervention) should include a physical examination, ECG, Chest X- rays, 2d echo and doppler, maximal exercise tolerance test and 24 hour ECG monitoring to assess:
1) presence and size of the residual VSD;
2) persistence of pulmonary hypertension;
3) presence of aortic regurgitation;
4) ventricular dimensions and function. Right or left ventriculotomy and/or the presence of a large surgical patch may impair ventricular function;
5) appearance of conduction disturbances or tachyarrhythmias.

If significant residual defects are absent and ventricular function is normal, operated patients can participate in moderate intensity sports. Selected cases with early primary correction through the right atrium can engage in high intensity sports.

Patent Ductus Arteriosus

Patent ductus arteriosus (PDA) is the persistence after birth of a normal fetal vessel that joins the aorta and the pulmonary artery. Normally it closes spontaneously by 4 days of age. Flow across the PDA (left to right shunt) depends on aorta and pulmonary pressures and on the diameter and length of the *ductus* itself.

A small PDA may be an occasional finding in an asymptomatic athlete. He presents a typical continuous murmur that is maximal at the second intercostal space inferior to the left clavicle.

ECG, Chest X-rays and echo show normal heart chamber dimensions the colour doppler can visualise the small turbulent flow in the pulmonary artery.

Athletes with a small PDA can participate in all competitive sports.

Patients with a moderate or large PDA present a louder continuous murmur often with thrill and bounding pulses due to widened systemic pulse pressure. Instrumental signs of left atrio-ventricular enlargement or combined hypertrophy and increased pulmonary blood flow are present. *Ductus* anatomy and size can be directly visualised with ECHO and the flow entity with colour doppler.

Closure of the PDA is indicated in these patients before sports practice and can be done either during cardiac catheterization occluding the *ductus* with coils or an umbrella device or by surgical operation.

3-6 months from the interventional or operative closure of the PDA patients can be evaluated for sports participation. If no significant residual shunt is detected, heart chamber dimensions are normalised and effort tolerance is normal, patients can engage in all competitive sports. When pulmonary hypertension is present it is necessary to wait for its normalisation before sports practice.

CHD with Obstruction to Ventricular Outflow

Pulmonary Stenosis

Right ventricular outflow obstruction can be localised at the level of the infundibulum, the valve or above the valve. Valvular pulmonary stenosis (PS) is the most common form and occurs in 7% of all CHD. The natural history and symptoms depend on the severity of the obstruction.

Athletes with mild PS (gradient <30 mmHg) or moderate PS (gradient 30-50mmHg) are generally asymptomatic but can be easily detected by an ejection click followed by a loud, rough systolic murmur best heard at the second left intercostal space.

Patients with severe PS (gradient >50 mmHg) may develop symptoms such as dyspnea, cyanosis and syncope during exercise. A second heart sound is widely split and the pulmonary component reduced. Right ventricular hypertrophy increases progressively with the increase of the gradient at ECG and

ECHO. Chest X-ray may often show a post-stenotic dilatation of the main and left pulmonary arteries, a right atrio-ventricular enlargement and in severe forms a decrease in pulmonary vascular markings and flow.

By 2d and Echo-doppler it is possible to localise the site of obstruction and assess the gradient. Tricuspid regurgitation helps to determine the right ventricular pressure.

Cardiac catheterization is indicated only when it is difficult to measure the flow velocity with doppler or in the moderate-severe forms in order to perform transluminal balloon valvuloplasty.

Recommendations

Patients with mild PS, no right ventricular hypertrophy and normal exercise tolerance test can participate in all competitive sports.

Patients with moderate PS should be evaluated individually in relation to the sport performed.

Severe forms should be corrected.

After correction (interventional cardiology or surgery) diagnostic studies and recommendations are the same as for pre-operative patients.

Pulmonary regurgitation is frequent after correction of PS but a mild to moderate grade of regurgitation does not controindicate sports practice. Yearly assessment with ECHO and a maximal exercise tolerance test is necessary.

Aortic Stenosis

The obstruction to left ventricular outflow may be localised in the subvalvular (20%), valvular (75%) or supravalvular region (5%). Congenital valvular aortic stenosis (AS) represents 6% of all CHD and is more common in males than in females. The valve is often the bicuspid and the turbulent flow promotes thickening of the cusps and so the obstruction tends to be progressive. Aortic regurgitation is sometimes prevalent in patients with bicuspid valve. Aortic coarctation may be associated and therefore the femoral pulses should always be checked.

Symptoms depend on the severity of the obstruction and are commonly absent in mild (gradient<20 mmHg) or moderate (<50 mmHg) stenosis. In severe forms (>50 mmHg) dyspnea, chest pain, easy fatigability, dizziness and syncope may occur during exercise. Occurrence of these symptoms in a athlete should alert the physician.

Physical examination reveals a left ventricular thrust at the apex and a systolic thrill at the right base, suprasternal notch and both carotid arteries in moderate-severe disease. A systolic click at the apex precedes a rough systolic murmur loudest at the first and second intercostal spaces and its grade correlates with the severity of stenosis.

ECG is normal in mild AS. Patients with severe obstruction demonstrate evidence of left ventricular hypertrophy and left ventricular strain, but in 25% of subjects the ECG may be normal.

Chest X-ray indicates dilation of the ascending aorta.

2D-ECHO shows left ventricular hypertrophy and bicuspid valve. Doppler can accurately predict transvalvular gradients (apical and suprasternal projection) and possibly associated aortic regurgitation.

Recommendations

Patients with a mild AS (< 20 mmHg) or isolated bicuspid aortic valve can participate in all competitive sports if the following criteria are met:
- absence of left ventricular hypertrophy (ECG-ECHO);
- normal exercise tolerance test (normal increase of blood pressure, no arrhythmia and absence of ischemic ST changes during exercise);
- normal systolic and diastolic left ventricular function;
- no arrhythmia on 24 hour ECG monitoring (also during training).

The patients with moderate to severe aortic stenosis cannot engage in competitive sports due to the risk of sudden death during exercise.

Yearly assessment with ECG, Echo-doppler, exercise testing and Holter ECG Monitoring is important in athletes at risk of AS progression.

Surgical repair or percutaneous balloon valvuloplasty should be considered in patients with symptoms, a large resting gradient (60-80 mmHg), or signs of left ventricular strain at rest or during exercise.

Discrete membranous subvalvular aortic stenosis consists of a membranous or fibrous ring just below the aortic valve. The findings are essentially the same as those of valvular AS and differentiating points are the absence of an aortic ejection click and the lower position of the systolic murmur. A diastolic murmur of aortic insufficiency is often heard.

Surgical correction is indicated also in asymptomatic mild subvalvular AS due to the risk of damage of the aortic valve by the jet.

Supravalvular aortic stenosis is a constriction of the ascending aorta just above the coronary the arteries. It is often associated with typical elfin faces and mental retardation (Williams syndrome) and therefore these patients do not practice competitive sports. The systolic thrill and murmur are typically best heard in the suprasternal notch and along the carotids. A difference in pulses and blood pressure between the right and left arm may be found, with the more prominent pulse and pressure being in the right arm.

With Echo-doppler it is possible to define the site, type and entity of the obstruction.

The criteria for sports practice are the same as applied for valvular AS.

After correction a variable degree of residual AS or regurgitation may be present. Non-invasive re-evaluation after 3-6 months is the same as for the unoperated athlete. Selected patients with a trivial gradient or regurgitation and regression of the left ventricular hypertrophy can engage in low/moderate intensity sports; yearly re-evaluation is necessary.

Coarctation of the Aorta

Coarctation of the aorta (CoAo) is a common cardiac abnormality (6% of CHD) characterised by an obstruction in the juxtaductal portion of the thoracic descending aorta. Most children and adolescents with CoAo are asymptomatic and participate in competitive sports with good results.

Diagnosis is often by chance and should be suspected in every athlete with:
1) diminution or absence of femoral pulses;
2) increase of arterial systolic pressure in the upper limbs with relatively lower pressure in the lower limbs;
3) mid-systolic blowing 2/6 murmur best heard in the interscapular area.

Severity may be assessed by the arm to leg blood pressure gradient but collateral vessels can reduce the gradient.

Chest X-ray may show notching of the ribs caused by dilated intercostal collaterals, ECG may show slight left ventricular hypertrophy. 2D-ECHO may directly visualise the CoAo and Colour-doppler reveals a flow disturbance and a high velocity jet at the site of obstruction providing a reasonable estimate of the CoAo pressure gradient.

All patients except those with mild CoAo should be corrected surgically or with balloon dilatation.

Recommendations

Athletes with mild CoAo (gradient<20 mmHG) and absence of arterial hypertension, large collateral vessels, LV hypertrophy, aortic root dilatation; with normal LV function and normal exercise testing results (including peak systolic blood pressure<230 mmHg) can participate in sports with moderate dynamic and low static demand. Sports with a danger of body collision should be avoided.

Moderate to severe CoAo (gradient>20 mmHg at rest) should be corrected.

Six months after correction the athlete can be re-evaluated using the same criteria followed for mild CoAo. In patients corrected with balloon angioplasty, an MRI can be useful to determine whether an aortic aneurysm is present.

Complex Congenital Heart Disease

Patients with complex CHD are generally cyanotic and do not participate in sports due to exercise intolerance and progressive hypoxemia. The same problem remains after palliative surgery.

Postoperative Tetralogy of Fallot

Corrective surgery (closure of VSD and right ventricular outflow tract enlargement) is generally performed in childhood. Most patients operated with good results are asymptomatic and present minimal pulmonary stenosis, mild to moderate pulmonary regurgitation and moderate right ventricular enlargement.

However, patients with operated tetralogy have a higher incidence of ventricular arrhythmias and sudden death that is impossible to forecast even with a complete cardiac evaluation. Competitive sports are therefore not recommended for these subjects.

Transposition of Great Arteries

a) Post Operative Mustard or Senning Operation
Patients with atrial repair of TGA even if asymptomatic have significant residual haemodynamic abnormalities (systemic right ventricle) and a higher incidence of arrhythmias. They can only participate in low intensity, dynamic, non competitive sports after complete non invasive evaluation.

b) Post Operative Arterial Switch
Patients with neonatal anatomic correction should have a better ventricular function and lower incidence of arrhythmias. However, actual exercise data and long-term results are limited for a reliable evaluation of sport fitness.

Potential post-operative sequelae that should be controlled are pulmonary stenosis, aortic regurgitation and stenosis or chinking of coronary arteries.

Postoperative Fontan Operation

This operation is performed for long-term palliation of patients with tricuspid atresia or single ventricle and is characterised by a direct communication from the venae cavae or right atrium to the pulmonary artery without a right sided pumping chamber. Exercise capacity remains limited due to reduced cardiac output and dangerous arrhythmias are frequent, so these patients can perform only non competitive, low intensity sports after complete non invasive evaluation.

Congenitally Corrected Transposition of Great Arteries

This anomaly is characterised by right position of the anatomical left ventricle which connects the right atrium to a posterior pulmonary artery. The anatomical right ventricle lies on the left and connects the left atrium to an anterior aorta so that blood circulation is functionally correct. Associated defects such as VSD, PS or systemic atrio-ventricular valve (tricuspid) abnormalities like the Ebstein anomaly are frequent and preclude participation in sports in many circumstances. Patients with CCTGA have an higher incidence of supraventricular tachycardia and late complete AV block.

Athletes with isolated CCTGA may be asymptomatic and the only physical finding is a single louder second heart sound. ECG may provide important clues to diagnosis with first degree AV block in 50% of patients and absence of Q waves in left precordial leads (inversion of septal depolarisation). Chest X-ray reveals the absence of the normal pulmonary artery segment and a smooth convexity of the left supracardiac border produced by the displaced aorta. 2D ECHO shows the ventricular inversion and great artery transposition.

Recommendations

Patients who have CCTGA without associated defects after evaluation with ECHO, exercise stress test and ambulatory ECG monitoring may participate in low intensity sports, better non competitive. Frequent periodic re-evaluation is necessary due to the risk of deterioration in systemic ventricular function (right ventricle), appearance of systemic AV valve (tricuspid valve) regurgitation and development of arrhythmias.

Ebstein Anomaly

A rare abnormality consisting of downward displacement of the tricuspid valve so that the septal leaflet is attached to the ventricular wall rather than to the fibrous ring. There is a wide spectrum in the haemodynamic severity of this malformation but also mild cases, often asymptomatic, have an increased risk of supraventricular tachyarrhythmias for the presence of WPW preexicitation.

ECG most often shows giant P waves, a prolonged PR interval and a variable degree of right bundle branch block or WPW pattern almost always type B resembling left bundle branch block.

ECHO permits the identification of displacement of the tricuspid leaflet and quantification of tricuspid regurgitation if present.

Recommendations

Athletes with a mild form of Ebstein anomaly with normal heart size, no evidence of arrhythmias on ambulatory ECG monitoring and normal exercise testing can participate in low-moderate intensity sports.

Congenital Coronary Anomalies

Congenital anomalies of coronary circulation are a rare and heterogeneous group of malformations with a high risk of sudden death during exercise. These anomalies should be suspected in athletes with syncope or dangerous arrhythmias during effort and can be divided in 3 types:

1) anomalous origin of left main coronary from the pulmonary trunk sometimes associated with myocardial infarction. A continuous murmur and ischemic ECG alterations are generally present. 2D-ECHO with colour-doppler can visualise the anomalous flow in the pulmonary artery.

2) anomalous origin of a coronary artery from a different aortic sinus. When the left coronary artery arises from the right sinus or the right coronary artery from the left sinus the course of the anomalous artery is between aorta and pulmonary trunk. During exertion the expansion of the great arteries may compress the anomalous coronary artery causing myocardial ischemia and sometimes sudden death. ECHO can identify the anomalous origin and course of coronary arteries and exercise testing may reveal ischemia but the diagnosis should be confirmed by selective coronary angiography.

3) coronary fistulas can be identified for a continuous murmur in the precordial area in an asymptomatic athlete. Myocardial ischemia may be present on ECG and ECHO with colour-doppler may detect enlarged coronary artery and the entrance site of the shunt which is characterised by a continuous turbulent flow pattern.

Recommendations

Detection of coronary anomaly with myocardial ischemia should result in exclusion from sports participation.

6 months from successful surgical or interventional correction if no ischemia or arrhythmias are present during exercise testing, participation in competitive sports of moderate intensity may be allowed.

Marfan Syndrome

The Marfan syndrome is a generalised disorder of connective tissue with characteristic skeletal, cardiac and ocular features. Long limbs and digits, tall stature, thoracic cage deformity, kyphoscoliosis and dislocation of the ocular lens are typical signs. The cardiovascular manifestations are mitral valve prolapse and aortic dilation with an increased risk of mitral and aortic regurgitation and aortic dissection. Cases of sudden death for aortic dissection have been reported in competitive athletes.

Diagnosis is suspected in tall stature athletes from skeletal features and should be confirmed with family history, eye examination and ECHO.

Recommendations

Patients with Marfan syndrome without aortic dilation or mitral regurgitation can participate in low static, moderate dynamic, non competitive sports without danger of body collision. Every 6 months aortic root dimensions should be verified by ECHO for the risk of progressive dilation.

Selected References

1. Colonna PL, Zeppilli P (1995) Cardiopatie congenite e sport. In: Zeppilli P ed. Cardiologia dello Sport. Roma CESI 369-393

2. Graham TP, Bricker JT, James FW, Strong WB (1994) Task Force 1: Congenital Heart Disease. 26th Bethesda Conference: Recommendations for determining eligibility for competition in athletes with cardiovascular abnormalities. J Am Coll Cardiol 24:867-873

3. COCIS (1996) Protocolli cardiologici per il giudizio di idoneita' allo sport agonistico Med Sport, 49:1-35

4. Calzolari A, Colonna PL, Dall'Olio M, De Luca NM, Drago F, Montella S, Picchio FM, Vignati G (1993) L'attività fisica nel bambino e nell'adolescente cardiopatico: criteri di valutazione clinica e certificazioni. Atti del gruppo di studio della Società Italiana di Cardiologia Pediatrica. Padova pag 1-25

5. Sklansky MS, Bricker JT (1993) Guidelines for exercise and sport partecipation in children and adolescents with congenital heart disease. Prog Pediatr Cardiol 2:55-66

6. Friedman WF (1992) Congenital heart disease in infancy and childhood. In: Braunwald E (ed) Heart Disease. W.B.Saunders Co Philadelphia, pp 887-956

7. Perloff JK. Congenital heart disease in adults.Heart Disease. W.B.Saunders Co Philadelphia, pp 966-991

8. Cullen S, Celermajer DS, Deanfield J (1991) Exercise in congenital heart disease Cardiol Young 1:129-135

9. Perrault H, Orblik SP (1989) Exercise after surgical repair of congenital cardiac lesions. Sports Medicine 7:18

10. Fratellone PM, Steinfeld L, Coplan N (1994) Exercise and congenital heart disease. Am Heart J 127:1676-1680

11. Cecconi M, Colonna PL, Bettuzzi MG, Manfrin M, Cesari GP et al (1991) Attività sportiva agonistica in soggetti sottoposti a correzione chirurgica di difetto interatriale tipo ostium secundum: esperienza su 9 casi. G Ital Cardiol 21:175-181

12. Wilmshurst PT, Byrne JC, Webb-People MM (1989) Relation between interatrial shunts and decompression sickness in divers. Lancet 2:1302-1306

13. Mori F, Favilli S, Zuppiroli A et al (1993) Idoneità sportiva in pazienti operati di coartazione aortica: valutazione mediante ecocardiografia Doppler da sforzo. G Ital Cardiol 23:225-230

14. Taylor AJ, Rogan KM, Virmani R (1992) Sudden cardiac death associated with isolated congenital coronary artery anomalies . J Am Coll Cardiol 20:640-646

15. Pelliccia A, Spataro A, Maron BJ (1993) Prospective echocardiographic screening for coronary artery anomalies in 1360 elite competitive athletes. Am J Cardiol 72:978-984

16. Pyeritz RE, Mc Kusick VA (1979) The Marfan syndrome: diagnosis and management. N Engl J Med 300:772-777

17. Colonna PL, Baldinelli A, Bucari S (1995) Sindrome di Marfan. In: Marino B, Dallapiccola B, Mastroiacovo P eds; Cardiopatie congenite e sindromi genetiche. Milano McGraw-Hill Libri Italia pag 85-98

Mitral Valve Prolapse: Criteria of Prognostic Evaluation in Athletes

P. Zeppilli, F. Caretta

Post-Graduate School of Sports Medicine, Catholic University, Rome, Italy

Definition, Etiology and Epidemiology

Mitral valve prolapse (MVP) is said to exist when a leaflet(s) or its portion protrudes abnormally above the annular plane. In the large majority of cases no definite causes of this abnormality can be identified (primary or idiopathic MVP), but in a minority of persons MVP is due to an identifiable etiology (secondary prolapse) such as rheumatic fever, ischemia or infarction, cardiomyopathies and connective tissue disorders [1, 2].

MVP occurs in 90 percent of subjects with Marfan syndrome [3] but, due to the rarity of this disease, they contribute to a very small part of the MVP population. A larger but less defined MVP group with some features of an inherited connective tissue disorder, especially pectus excavatum [4, 5], has been identified and awaits further studies to clarify the genetic abnormalities responsible and the patterns of its inheritance. Present data suggest significant family aggregation consistent with polygenic inheritance; the likelihood of a first degree relative having MVP is about two and half times the normal population average [4].

Primary MVP is probably the most frequent valvular anomaly in the clinical practice [6]. Auscultatory and/or echocardiographic signs of MVP occurs in about 4-6% of the general population, with a larger prevalence in females and in subjects with a thin body habitus [7-11]. A slightly higher prevalence has been reported in the pediatric population which indirectly confirms the "congenital" origin theory of the disease [12, 13].

A prevalence (3.2%) similar to that observed in the general population has been reported in a large cohort of top-ranking sportsmen seen at the Sports Science Institute of Rome [14]. However, MVP can be found in 20-30 percent of male and female athletes, characterized by tall height and thin body habitus such as basket and volleyball players [15, 16]. Such prevalence is very close to that found at the Montreal Olympic Games in 1976 (22%) [17].

Most individuals and athletes with MVP are asymptomatic. At the other extreme, patients with severe MVP often have symptoms and signs related to valve dysfunction and progressive regurgitation. However, some subjects have symptoms such as chest pain, dyspnea, fatigue, poor exercise tolerance, palpitation, orthostatic hypotension, syncope and presyncope which cannot be explained on the basis of the presence and severity of mitral valve abnormality alone.

The pathogenesis of these symptoms appears to be related to metabolic-neuroendocrine abnormalities (MVP syndrome) [18].

Asymptomatic athletes with minor degrees of prolapse usually have no risk of deterioration. In these subjects, MVP should be considered a normal variant of valve motion and therefore restriction of physical activity (for fear of medical complications for the athlete or legal problems for the physician) is rarely justified. On the other hand, adverse outcome may occur in a small subset of subjects who suffer complications such as severe mitral regurgitation, infective endocarditis, cerebral transitory ischemic attacks or strokes [19, 20], life-threatening arrhythmias and, very rarely, sudden death [1, 2]. The main goal of sports cardiologists is thus to identify such subjects before complications arise.

Diagnostic Criteria

Standardized and critical diagnostic criteria are interventions of first choice. The diagnosis can be made on the basis of the typical auscultatory hallmarks, i.e. mid to late systolic click and murmur, but today echocardiography (ECHO) also plays an essential role.

It is universally accepted that ECHO criteria must be selective to avoid an excessive number of false positive diagnosis [21] especially in the absence of the characteristic auscultatory findings (silent prolapse). Presently, major and minor diagnostic criteria for prolapse are considered [22]:
● major criteria include late systolic posterior displacement on M-mode, bowing of mitral leaflets into the left atrium on the two-dimensional (2D) parasternal long-axis view and thickening and redundancy of leaflets;
● minor criteria include holosystolic posterior displacement ("hammock-like" pattern) on M-mode, bowing of the mitral leaflets into the left atrium on 2D apical views and isolate late systolic mitral regurgitation on ECHO Doppler and Color-Doppler [23, 24]. Minor degrees of bowing in the apical views may be a normal variant of mitral valve motion due to the nonplanar shape of the annulus in the region of the anterior leaflet attachment [25].

Any of the major criteria should be sufficient for the diagnosis while minor criteria should suggest but not definitively prove MVP, although they become more important when symptoms, ST-T wave abnormalities, arrhythmias and conduction disturbances are present. Since left ventricular enlargement following training may mask MVP, ECHO examination performed after an adequate period of detraining may be helpful in athletes with inexplicable symptoms or marked ECG abnormalities but without apparent signs of prolapse.

ECHO-Doppler is not only the keystone of the diagnosis but is very helpful to assess prognosis and serves as a baseline for future controls. The degree of thickening and redundancy and the presence and extent of mitral regurgitation significantly influence outcome. Subjects with severe leaflet redundancy and mitral annular enlargement at first examination have a significantly higher probability of undergoing progressive mitral regurgitation. Acute mitral insufficiency may also occur in these patients as consequence of chordal rupture, causing failure of coaptation of the two leaflets and slipping of the flail portion into the left atrium (flail mitral valve) [26, 27]. Today, transesophageal ECHO can accurately assess flail leaflets and possible associated vegetations due to infective endocarditis [28, 29]. Transesophageal ECHO is also very helpful in identifying potential sources of systemic emboli within the left atrium and therefore it may be desirable in this subset of patients [30, 31].

Sports Eligibility

In Italy preparticipation screening and periodic reevaluation of athletes for medical certification of fitness for competitive sports are required by law.

Therefore, selective diagnostic criteria must be adopted in young, usually asymptomatic, MVP athletes to avoid unnecessary restriction of sports activity but, on the other hand, early identification of high-risk subjects is mandatory. Presently, because of the high short-term risk of sports requiring moderate to maximum physical efforts and cardiovascular involvement, we think that MVP athletes with one or more of the following conditions should be excluded from competitions:
1) Marfan syndrome, because of the high risk of mitral valve deterioration and sudden death due to aortic rupture;
2) severe mitral regurgitation, marked leaflets redundancy associated with moderate regurgitation, combined tricuspid and aortic prolapse and regurgitation (mixomatous disease);
3) high-risk ventricular arrhythmias, especially when associated with prolonged QTc interval and electrophysiological signs of electrical instability. There is now strong evidence that life-threatening ventricular arrhythmias and sudden death in MVP patients are frequently due to underlying, often occult, pathologic substrate different from MVP such as arrhythmogenic right ventricular dysplasia, myocarditis, etc. [32-35]. This can explain the high prevalence of ventricular late potentials found in MVP patients with complex arrhythmias [36] and indicates the need to search for other arrhythmogenic substrates particularly when ventricular premature beats do not have the typical QRS morphology (right bundle branch block);
4) effort-induced supraventricular tachycardia or atrial fibrillation, especially when associated with cardiac preexcitation;
5) frequent and/or prolonged episodes of typical and atypical chest pain, especially when effort-induced;
6) unexplained syncope or presyncope.
The prognostic significance in athletes of some other aspects of MVP syndrome such as repolarization abnormalities, high degree bradyarrhyhmias and atrioventricular conduction disturbances, orthostatic hypotension, vasovagal syncope or presyncope is still unclear. These findings do not necessarily have

pathological significance and do not *per se* implicate disqualification form sports. They should be interpreted in the athlete's clinical context and in many cases accurate long-term follow-up studies can help to resolve controversial aspects of this problem. The frequency of clinical and ECHO follow-up should be determined by the initial presentation. When mitral regurgitation is present, one should carefully follow left atrial and left ventricular size and function.

Prophylactic interventions are necessary to avoid the risk of a disabling infective endocarditis in the subset of subjects at higher risk due to valve redundancy, flail leaflet, moderate to severe mitral regurgitation, etc. However, it should be emphasized that probably the most important therapeutic approach in MVP subjects and athletes is to explain the mechanisms of symptoms and to reassure them.

References

1. Barlow JB (1992) Idiopathic (degenerative) and rheumatic mitral valve prolapse: historical aspects and overview. J Heart Valve Dis 1:163
2. Shah PM (1992) Mitral valve prolapse - The elusive definitions and differing criteria of diagnosis. J Heart Valve Dis 1:160
3. Hirata K, Triposkiadis F, Sparks E, et al (1992) The Marfan syndrome: cardiovascular physical findings and diagnostic correlates. Am Heart J 123 (3):743
4. Wilcken DE (1992) Genes, gender and geometry and the prolapsing mitral valve. Aust N Z J Med. 22 (Suppl 5):556
5. Seliem MA, Duffy CE, Gidding SS, Berdusis K, Benson DW Jr (1992) Echocardiographic evaluation of the aortic root and mitral valve in children and adolescents with isolated pectus excavatum: comparison with Marfan patients. Pediatr Cardiol 13:20
6. Roberts WC (1984) The 2 most common congenital heart diseases (Editorial). Am J Cardiol 53:1198
7. Procacci PM, Savran SV, Schreiter SL et al (1976) Prevalence of clinical mitral-valve prolapse in 1169 young women. N Engl J Med 294:1086
8. Rizzon P, Biasco G, Brindicci G, et al (1979) Prolasso della valvola mitrale: epidemiologia e criteri diagnostici. Atti del Congresso della Società Italiana di Cardiologia 1979. G Ital Cardiol :(Suppl. 1) (abstract)
9. Savage DD, Devereux RB, Garrison RJ et al (1983) Mitral valve prolapse in the general population. 2. Clinical features: the Framingham study. Am Heart J 106:577
10. Zuppiroli A, Favilli S, Risoli A, et al (1990) Il prolasso della valvola mitrale: studio della prevalenza mediante ecocardiografia bidimensionale in una popolazione giovanile. G Ital Cardiol 20:161
11. Gemelli A, Marilungo M, De Ruvo S, et al (1992) Mitral valve prolapse. Age and sex incidence echocardiographic diagnosis and clinical and electrocardiographic correlations. Minerva Med 83 (1-2):9
12. Gupta R, Jain BK, Gupta HP, et al (1992) Mitral valve prolapse: two dimensional echocardiography revals a high prevalence in three to twelve year old children. Indian Pediatr 29:415
13. Arfken CL, Schulman P, McLaren MJ, Lachman AS (1993) Mitral valve prolapse and body habitus in children. Pediatr Cardiol 14:33

14. Spataro A, Pelliccia A, Caselli G, et al (1989) Utility of routinary echocardiography in the screening of a large population of top-level athletes. In: Lubich T, Venerando A, Zeppilli P. eds. Sports Cardiology II. Aulo Gaggi ed. pag. 367

15. Vannicelli R, Cameli S, Corsetti R, et al (1995) Physiological and clinical aspects of the cardiovascular system in volleyball players. Proceedings of the IIIrd Symposium of Sport Medicine Applied to Volleyball, Paris, October (in press)

16. Aspromonte N, Tranquilli C, Cecchetti F, et al (1984) Profilo cardiologico clinico e strumentale di giocatrici di basket di elevato livello. Med Sport. 37:293

17. Laurenceau JL, Turcot J, Dusmenil JG (1980) Echocardiographic study of olympic athletes. In: Lubich T, Venerando A. eds. Sports Cardiology. Aulo Gaggi ed. (abstract) pag. 705

18. Boudoulas H (1992) Mitral valve prolapse: etiology, clinical presentation and neuroendocrine function. J Heart Valve Dis 1(2):175

19. Jones HR Jr, Naggar CZ, Seljan MP, et al (1982) Mitral valve prolapse and cerebral ischemic events: a comparison between a neurology population with stroke and a cardiology population with mitral valve prolapse observed for five years. Stroke 13:451

20. Giovannoni G, Fritz VU (1993) Transient ischemic attacks in younger and older patients. A comparative study of 798 patients in South Africa. Stroke 24:947

21. Zeppilli P (1981) Il prolasso della valvola mitrale nella popolazione sportiva: epidemiologia, profilassi e terapia di una pandemia. G Ital Cardiol 11:1800

22. Feigenbaum H (1991) Echocardiography in the management of mitral valve prolapse. Aust NZ J Med 22:550

23. Miyatake K, Izumi S, Okamoto M et al (1986) Semiquantitative grading of severity of mitral regurgitation by real time two-dimensional doppler flow imaging technique. J Am Coll Cardiol 7:82

24. Pennestri F, Loperfido F (1991) Ecocardiografia Doppler. Galeno ed. Perugia pag. 133

25. Levine RA, Triulzi MO, Harrigan P, et al (1987) The relationship of mitral annular shape to the diagnosis of mitral valve prolapse. Circulation 75:756

26. Ballester M, Foale R, Presbitero P, et al (1983) Cross-sectional echocardiographic features of ruptured chordae tendine. Eur Heart J 4:795

27. Pearson AC, Vrain J, Mrosek D, Labovitz AJ (1990) Color Doppler echocardiographic evaluation of patients with a flail mitral leaflet. J Am Coll Cardiol 16:232

28. Hozumi T, Yoshikawa J, Yoshida K, et al (1990) Direct visualization of ruptured chordae tendineae by transesophageal echocardiography. J Am Coll Cardiol 16:1315

29. Himelman RB, Kusumoto F, Oken K, et a (1991) The flail mitral valve: echocardiographic findings by precordial and transesophageal imaging and Doppler Color flow mapping. J Am Coll Cardiol 17:272

30. Labovitz AJ, Camp A, Castello R, et al (1993) Usefulness of transesophageal echocardiography in unexplained cerebral ischemia. Am J Cardiol 72:1448

31. Espinola-Zavaleta N, Vargas-Barron J, Romero-Cardenas A, et al (1993) Transthoracic and transesophageal echocardiography in the study of young adults with a cerebral ischemic event. Arch Inst Cardiol Mex 63:311

32. Bharati S, Granston AS, Liebston PR, et al (1981) The conduction system in mitral valve prolapse syndrome and sudden death. Am Heart J 101:667

33. Boudoulas H, Schaal SF, Stang JM, et al (1990) Mitral valve prolapse: cardiac arrest with long-term survival. Int J Cardiol 26:37

34. Farb A, Tang AL, Atkinson JB, McCarthy WF, Virmani R (1992) Comparison of car-

diac findings in patients with mitral valve prolapse who die suddenly to those with fatal noncardiac conditions. Am J Cardiol 70 (2):234

35. Corrado D, Thiene G, Basso C, Rossi L, Nava A (1993) Arrhythmogenic subtrates in juvenile sudden death from mitral valve prolapse."The New Frontiers of Arrhythmias" IX:3:597

36. Leclerq JF, Malergue MC, Coumel P (1993) Late potentials and mitral valve prolapse. Arch Mal Coeur Vaiss 86:285

Cardiomyopathies, Myocarditis and Sport

A. Nava, A. Corrado, L. Oselladore

Department of Cardiology, University of Padua, Medical School, Padua, Italy

Cardiomyopathies and myocarditis are very important in athletics because they cause ventricular arrhythmias and juvenile sudden death [1].

A very precise study performed in the Veneto Region (situated in North East Italy) showed that these pathologies are the main cardiac cause of sudden death in young people. In a series of 207 cases collected over 16 years, 71 patients were affected with these pathologies (30%), versus 66 patients with coronary disease, 24 with mitral valve prolapse and 22 with defects of the conduction system. This percentage tends to increase if we consider that about 50% of patients affected with mitral valve prolapse also had right ventricular pathology undiagnosed during life [2, 3].

Among these 71 cases arrhythmogenic right ventricular cardiomyopathy (ARVC) was the most frequent disease (27 cases), see Table 1.

In sports medicine the problems caused by these diseases are completely different from the problems usually seen in clinical practice and are exclusively related to the possibility, or not, of performing sports activity. In sports medicine only borderline cases where diagnosis is more difficult are usually found.

Table 1. Target project of Juvenile Sudden Death, Veneto, Italy

Cardiomyopathies and myocarditis (71 cases)	
Right ventricular cardiomyopathy	= 27 cases
Myocarditis	= 20 cases
Hypertrophic cardiomyopathy	= 14 cases
Dilated cardiomyopathy	= 10 cases

Arrhythmogenic Right Ventricular Cardiomyopathy

ARVC is a frequent cause of juvenile sudden death of unknown etiology, and has recently become of interest in sports medicine. This cardiomyopathy prevalently involves the right ventricle and is characterized by progressive myocardial atrophy. The disease is not due to abnormal development of the right ventricle as previously thought but rather to a progressive necrotic myocellular process. Necrotic tissue is substituted by adipose and fibrous tissue in different percentages from case to case [4].

The pathology proceeds from the epicardium to the endocardium and in about 30% of patients the left ventricle is also involved later on. The fibrous-fatty substitution can be diffuse but very often the pathological process is segmentary, mainly involving one to three areas of the right ventricle (apex, inflow tract, outflow tract); in other cases, however, the process can be widespread. The main clinical outcome is electrical instability. Heart failure is a rare event which appears only when the myocardial fibro-fatty substitution is massive [5].

The electrophysiological mechanisms generating arrhythmias are multiple: reentry is the most common and appears because the pathologic process creates many reentry circuits, constituted by healthy fibers separated by fibro-fatty areas. Enhanced automaticity and trigger activity are other causes of electrical instability, probably underestimated and appearing during physical activity. These arrhythmias could be the main cause of juvenile sudden death [6, 7].

Numerous causes are implicated in provoking this type of electrical instability. Increased reflex sympathetic tone due to the distruction of right ventricular epicardial sympathetic receptors is the first cause. The second is the acute phase of the disease. In this situation necrosis is present in different areas of the heart and the clinical outcome is very similar to myocarditis. The third cause is the alternate healthy and diseased myocardial areas which generate an important QT dispersion due to a dishomogeneous cardiac activation and repolarization. Finally, the progression of the disease caused by successive episodes of acute myocyte death tends to change the electrical instability over time.

The incidence of the disease is about 6/10.000 but it is probably underestimated. The disease appears in different forms depending on the extension of the pathology (extensive, moderate, mild) [5] (Table 2). An epidemiological study of the disease demonstrated that the massive form is present only in only 6-8% of cases, the moderate form in 35-40% and the mild form in 40-50%. Except for the massive form, right ventricular function is normal in the majority of cases and the affected subject can lead a normal life and participate in sports activities with good results. In these subjects the disease very often goes undiagnosed and dangerous arrhythmias could appear suddenly.

These data are in contrast with earlier studies in which patients with the massive form of the disease were prevalent. Today it has been demonstrated that morbidity is higher and symptoms and mortality less frequent than previously believed because many asymptomatic subjects are now diagnosed.

The etiology of myocardial atrophy has still not been clarified. At various times viral, toxic or autoimmune factors have been proposed.

A genetic hypothesis is under study at present. More than 40% of cases have a family history of the disease. Recent studies identified three different loci responsible for the disease on chromosomes 14, 1 and 2 respectively (8, 9 - personal data). These loci are close to others also coding for proteins found in the myocardium, such as alpha-actinin 1 and 2 [8].

Table 2. Diagnostic findings of ARVC

Mild Form

⇨   Clinical findings: normal life (sports activity), different ventricular arrhythmias (especially monomorphic arrhythmias of the infundibular tract), many asymptomatic subjects (60% of cases).

⇨   ECG: normal or slightly altered, late potentials present in 32% of cases, preferably with 80 hertz filters.

⇨   Echocardiography and angiography: normal or slightly increased RV end-diastolic volume, ejection fraction (EF) normal, one or more segmental kinetic alterations (subtricuspidal or apical bulging, infundibular pulmonary dilatation, disarrangement of trabecular pattern).

⇨   Normal coronaries.

Moderate Form

⇨   Clinical findings: different ventricular arrhythmias, good physical performance, rarely no arrhythmias.

⇨   ECG: T negative in V1-V2 or V1-V2-V3, late potential at signal-averaged ECG,

⇨   Echocardiography and angiography: RV moderately enlarged with end-diastolic volume between 80-139 ml/m². EF normal or slightly depressed, presence of numerous segmentary alterations of RV.

⇨   Normal coronaries.

Extensive Form

⇨   Clinical findings: symptoms are: sustained ventricular tachycardias, with left B.B.B. morphology, cardiomegaly, effort dyspnea, cyanosis, heart failure.

⇨   ECG: negative T wave in many precordial leads with epsilon waves, right atrial enlargement, low QRS voltage.

⇨   Echocardiography and angiography: right atrial enlargement, EF reduction with increased right ventricular end-diastolic volume (more than 140 ml/m²), RV enormously dilated with diffused hypokinesia.

⇨   Normal coronaries.

As in muscular dystrophy, it is possible that these patients present abnormalities of the myocellular structure which in particular situations, probably when unknown modulating factors appear, provoke myocitis necrosis. The necrotic process seems to be prevalent at a young age [10].

Diagnosis is clinical and based on the observation of typical arrhythmias, familiarity, ECG modifications (Fig. 1), demonstration of morphologic and functional abnormalities of the right ventricle at echography (Fig. 2), angiography or magnetic resonance, in the absence of other cardiac diseases. Endomyocardial biopsy is often necessary to confirm the diagnosis.

The disease has a typical clinical polymorphism due to the different extensions of the pathologic process. Thus, it is quite difficult to diagnose the minor forms of the disease which are usually characterized by cryptogenetic, apparently idiopathic, ventricular arrhythmias. It is these forms which prevalently concerns sports medicine.

It is important to underline that the disease can have a concealed asymptomatic phase. The asymptomatic phase could persist for the entire lifetime or

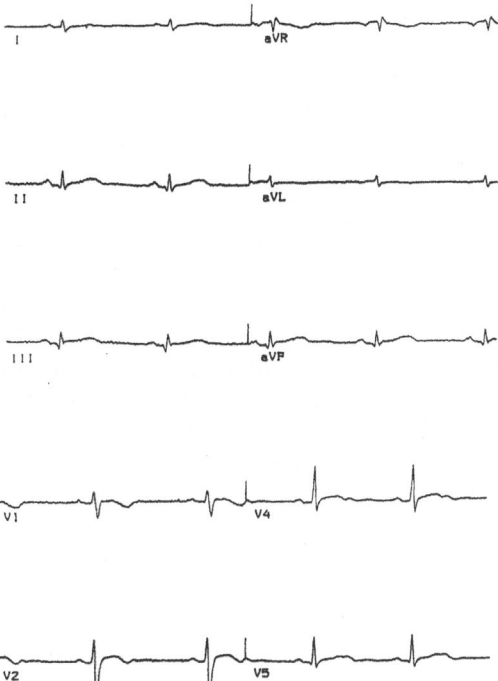

Fig. 1. B.P. 22 years. Familiar form of right ventricular cardiomyopathy. Basal ECG. Note T negative in L1-L2- L3 (V1-V2-V3) and diphasic in L4-L5 (V4-V5). The voltages of QRS are low and R is high in L1-L2-L3

may suddenly end. Furthermore, electrical instability can change in accordance with the progression of the disease causing the sudden appearance of severe and sometimes life-threatening ventricular arrhythmias.

The diagnostic criteria of the disease were recently published in the British Heart Journal by the Task Force on Arrhythmogenic Right Ventricular Cardiomyopathy of the European Society of Cardiology [11].

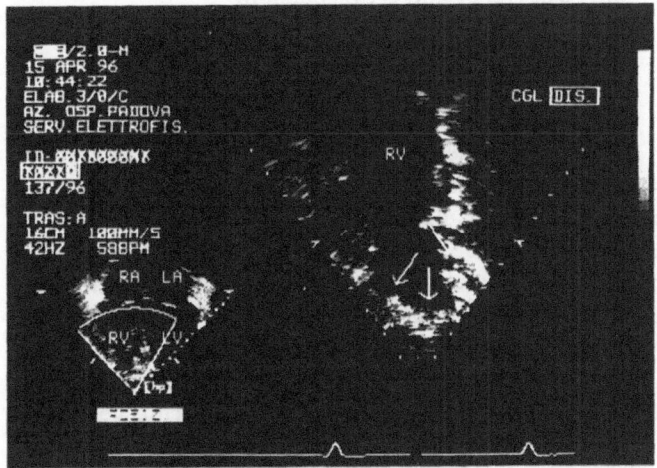

Fig. 2. G.P. 24 years. This subject experienced a sustained ventricular tachycardia during jogging. Brother died suddenly. Echocardiogram four chamber apical view. Note diskynesia with bulging of apical region of R.V.

Hypertrophic Cardiomyopathy

Hypertrophic cardiomyopathy has always been considered the most important myocardial disease as far as sports medicine is concerned [12, 13]. There are different reasons: it can cause sudden death and subjects are often asymptomatic and able to obtain high level athletic performances. In borderline cases it is very difficult to differentiate a pathologic from a physiologic hypertrophy, the latter being very common in athletes. This is a major issue concerning the diagnosis of the disease. In fact, once it has been assessed that a pathologic hypertrophy is present (expression of a minor form of hypertrophic cardiomyopathy) it is advisable to avoid competitive sports.

There is not complete agreement with this point of view as some Authors think that patients - asymptomatic and without inducible ventricular arrhythmias and so affected by minor forms of the disease - should be allowed to do competitive sports. This belief has to be criticized if we accept that the danger of the disease is not correlated with its severity.

In fact, one of the most important causes of sudden death in these subjects is the myocardial fibrosis present in the hypertrophic areas which provokes dishomogeneous ventricular activation. When this happens sympathetic stimulation and myocardial ischemia appearing during effort can trigger dangerous arrhythmias. These determining factors are not necessarily correlated with the severity of the hypertrophy.

Today modern diagnostic techniques make diagnosis easier. In the future genetic studies could also help diagnose borderline cases.

At present, a septal thickness of 16 mm is considered normal, in top-level athletes even if the population normal value is 12 mm. These are extreme conditions which should be considered normal only in the absence of other signs of the disease such as family history, abnormal ventricular filling at 2D and color-doppler echo-scan, systolic anterior movement of the mitral valve, giant T wave left ventricular hypertrophy or ST depression at ECG, severe ventricular arrhythmias, ST abnormalities at Holter and QT dispersion.

Myocarditis

Myocarditis [14] is not a rare cause of death during sports activity. However, the problem is not only to diagnose the disease but also to determine if a patient who had myocarditis is healed and if he can continue to play sports. Banal intercurrent feverish episodes can cause an inflammation of the myocardium. If the inflammatory process is focal a patient can be completely asymptomatic and continue playing sports because he does not know he is affected by the disease. Focal myocarditis can cause sudden death by inducing either a ventricular fibrillation or a paroxysmal complete A-V block if there is inflammation of the conduction system. Thus it is a cause of sudden death which is very difficult to predict. When fever is present focal myocarditis has to be suspected if the ST segment changes, A-V block, atrial or ventricular hyperkinetic arrhythmias appear on ECG and palpitations or dizziness are present. Fever may be the only symptom. Chest pain is not common and very often the ECG is normal. Widespread myocarditis is easy to diagnose and is characterized by heart failure, dyspnea, chest pain, heart enlargement at chest X-ray and a S-T segment elevation at ECG. Myocardial enzymes are increased. Acute focal myocarditis normally leads to a complete recovery. However, about 50% of the widespread forms evolve towards either a dilated cardiomyopathy or an incomplete recovery. Recovery must be complete to permit sports activity. An incomplete recovery with myocardial scars can allow a normal life but could be dangerous and provoke electrical instability. Judging complete recovery is often possible only after invasive diagnostic procedures such as endomyocardial biopsy to exclude the presence of necrotic areas with inflammatory infiltrates.

Dilated Cardiomyopathy

Dilated cardiomyopathy is less important as far as sports medicine is concerned. It is very rare in young people and when symptoms such as dyspnoea or palpitations appear, athletic performance decreases and the athlete undergoes a cardiological exam. The main problem is to differentiate the physiologic dilatation, frequent in athletes with a moderate reduction of the ejection fraction of the left ventricle, from an initial form of dilated cardiomyopathy. Electrocardiographic changes (atrial enlargement, left ventricular hypertrophy, left bundle branch block) and echocardiographic abnormalities (LVEDV > 100 ml/m, EF < 45%, M/V < 0.8, P/ESV < 2.5, ventricular filling abnormalities, widespread or localized kinetic abnormalities) (Table 3) are the qualifying points of a differential diagnosis [15].

Table 3. Main differential aspects of hypertrophic and dilated cardiomyopathy

	Dilated	Hypertrophic
Myocardial mass	$\uparrow \rightarrow \uparrow \uparrow$	$\uparrow \uparrow \uparrow$
Ventricular end diastolic volume	$\uparrow \uparrow \rightarrow \uparrow \uparrow \uparrow$	$\downarrow \downarrow \rightarrow$ normal
Atrial enlargement	+	++
Assymetric septal hypertrophy	0	+
Myocardial disarray	0	++
Intramural coronary path	0	+
Contractility	$\downarrow \downarrow \downarrow$	$\uparrow \uparrow \rightarrow \downarrow$
Abnormal ventricular filling	0	+++
Subaortic stenosis	0	0↔+
Mitral incompetence	+	++
Mitral valve pathologic movement	0	++
Intracavitary thrombosis	++	0

Another problem is to distinguish the idiopathic left bundle branch block of the young from the conduction block which can be the first sign of dilated cardiomyopathy. To prevent clinical manifestations of the disease that could be favored by physical activity it is important to diagnose the disease during the asymptomatic phase, which can prove to be quite difficult. In the future a better knowledge of the initial alteration present in the disease and genetic studies could favorably help diagnosis. Family history of dilated cardiomyopathy and ventricular localized kinetic abnormalities are often the only signs of the disease.

References

1. Corrado D, Thiene G, Nava A, Rossi L, Pennelli N (1990) Sudden death in young competitive athletes: clinicopathologic correlations in 22 cases. Am J Med 89:588-96
2. Basso C, Frescura C, Corrado D, Muriago M, Angelini A, Daliento L, Thiene G (1995) Congenital heart disease and sudden death in the young. Hum Path 26:1065-1072
3. Corrado D, Basso C, Poletti A, Angelini A, Valente M, Thiene G (1994) Sudden Death in theYoung: is Acute Coronary Thrombosis the Major Precipitating Factor? Circulation 90:2315-23
4. Thiene G, Nava A, Corrado D, Rossi L, Pennelli N (1988) Right ventricular cardiomyopathy and sudden death in young people. N Engl J Med 318:129-33
5. Nava A, Thiene G, Canciani B, Martini B, Daliento L, Buja GF, Fasoli G (1992) Clinical profile concealed form of arrhythmogenic right ventricular cardiomyopathy presenting with apparently idiopathic ventricular arrhythmias. Int J Cardiol 35:195-206
6. Oselladore L, Nava A, Buja G, Turrini P, Daliento L, Livolsi B, Thiene G (1995) Signal-averaged electrocardiography in familial form of arrhythmogenic right ventricular cardiomyopathy. Am J Cardiol 75:1038-1041
7. Corrado D, Nava A, Buja G, Martini B, Fasoli G, Oselladore L, Turrini P, Thiene G (1996) Familial cardiomyopathy underlies syndrome of right bundle branch block, ST segment elevation and sudden death. J Am Coll Cardiol
8. Rampazzo A, Nava A, Danieli GA, Buja GF, Daliento L, Fasoli G, Scorgnamiglio R, Corrado D, Thiene G (1994) The gene for arrhythmogenic right ventricular cardiomyopathy maps on chromosome 14q23-q24. Hum Molec Genet 3:959-962
9. Rampazzo A, Nava A, Erne P, Eberhard M, Vian E, Slomp P, Tiso N, Thiene G, Danieli GA (1995) A new locus for arrhythmogenic right ventricular cardiomyopathy (ARVD2) maps to chromosome 14q42-q43. Hum Molec Genet 4:2151-2154
10. Basso C, Thiene G, Corrado D, Angelini A, Nava A, Valente M (1996) Arrhythmogenic right ventricular cardiomyopathy. Dysplasia, dystrophy of myocarditis? Circulation 94:983-991
11. McKenna WJ, Thiene G, Nava A, Fontaliran F, Blomstrom-Lundqvist C, Fontaine G, Camerini F (1994) Diagnosis of arrhythmogenic right ventricular dysplasia/cardiomyopathy. Br Heart J 71:215-218
12. Maron BJ, Roberts WC, McAllister HA, Rosing DR, Epstein SE (1980) Sudden death in young athletes. Circulation 62:218-29
13. Maron BJ, Mitchell JH (1994) Revised Eligibility Recommendations for Competitive Athletes With Cardiovascular Abnormalities. J Am Coll Cardiol 24:848-50
14. Aretz HT, Billingham ME, Edwards WD, et al (1987) Myocarditis: a histopatologic

definition and classification. Am J Cardiovasc Pathol 1:3-14
15. Wynn J, Braunwald E (1992) The cardiomyopaties and myocarditis. In E. Braunwald: Heart Disease. A textbook of cardiovascular medicine. W.B. Saunders Company, Philadelphia

Pathology of Cardiac Diseases at Risk of Sudden Death in Athletes

D. Corrado, C. Basso, G.O. Thiene

Department of Pathology, University of Padua, Italy

Introduction

A structural cardiovascular abnormality is found at autopsy in most cases of sudden death in athletes [1-8]. The cause of sudden death reflects the age of partecipants. Atherosclerotic coronary artery disease is by far the most common cause of sudden death in athletes over 35 years of age [2, 4, 5], whereas a broader spectrum of pathologic conditions even including cardiomyopathies [3, 6, 7, 10], congenital coronary artery anomalies [11, 12], mitral valve prolapse [13], conduction system abnormalities [14], myocarditis [1, 5, 6] and aortic dissection [6, 7] may underlie sudden fatalities in younger athletes. The cardiovascular pathologic substrates are usually clinically silent and the cause of death found at autopsy had been not diagnosed or even suspected in over 75% of athletes who died suddenly [6, 7]. In addition, the low sensitivity of clinical tests in detecting such cardiovascular abnormalities may invalidate screening programs for prevention of sport-related fatalities [6, 7].

In this review we will discuss each cardiovascular condition at risk of sudden death during sports with particular reference to pathologic findings and pathophysiology of sudden cardiac arrest.

Atherosclerotic Coronary Artery Disease

Atherosclerotic coronary artery disease is the major cause of sudden death in adult and elderly exercising subjects. Most deaths occur in running, jogging, and long distance racing. Pathologic findings are consistent with an underlying severe and extensive atherosclerotic coronary artery disease, with two or more coronary trunks critically obstructed in over 70% of cases and frequently associated with post-infarction scars; often there is pathologic evidence of acute coronary thrombosis and acute myocardial infarction [1, 2, 4, 5, 15]. In accordance with these pathologic substates, pathophysiologic mechanisms of sudden cardiac arrest include either an ischemic-related electrical instability, which may be precipitated by an effort-induced increase of myocardial oxygen demand or by a fresh occlusive thrombosis [16], or a primary ventricular arrhythmia arising from a postinfarction myocardial scar. In these old sudden death victims, previous symptoms suggestive of the presence of coronary atheroslerosis have been often recognized and risk factors are frequently present, including hypertension, smoking and hypercholesterolaemia [17].

Atherosclerotic coronary artery disease is an important cause of sudden death even in young competitive athletes [6, 7, 18, 19]. Coronary atherosclerosis in the young exhibits distinctive pathologic features such as extent, site and morphology of the obstructive atherosclerotic plaques. In young athletes dying by coronary artery disease in the absence of previous angina pectoris and/or myocardial infarction, sudden death is frequently the first manifestation of the disease, [7, 18]. Coronary atherosclerosis is more often a "single-vessel disease" that affect the left anterior descending coronary artery; obstructive plaques are not complicated by acute thrombosis and are mostly fibrocellular due to a neointimal smooth muscle cell hyperplasia in the presence of a preserved tunica media [19]. These morphologic features have been suggested to underlie abnormal hypervasoreactivity and possibly precipitate arrhythmic cardiac arrest by vasospastic myocardial ischemia [19]. The in vivo identification of these young athletes at risk of ischemic cardiac arrest is a challenge, due to the absence of risk factors and warning symptoms as well as the limitations of stress tests in detecting myocardial ischemia.

Cardiomyopathies

Hypertrophic Cardiomyopathy

Hypertrophic cardiomyopathy (HCM) is a heart muscle disease, usually genetically trasmitted and characterized by a hypertrophied, non dilated left ventricle in the absence of predisposing diseases [3, 9]. The familial form of HCM is genetically heterogeneous and a number of mutations encoding for contractile proteins such as beta myosin heavy chain, cardiac troponin T and alpha-tropomyosin have been identified [20, 21]. The disease has been implicated as the principal cause of sudden cardiac arrest on the athletic field in the USA [3, 6]. Up to 50% of sport-related cardiac fatalities were attributed to HCM by Maron et al [3]. Gross pathologic features include 1) cardiomegaly due to left ventricular hypertrophy which is usually "asymmetric" with disproportionate septal tickening (septum/left ventricular free wall thickness > 1.3) (Fig. 1A); 2) reduction in left ventricular chamber size with increased myocardial "stiffness" which may critically impair diastolic compliance and intramural coronary blood filling; 3) a subaortic septal plaque associated with a thickening of the anterior leaflet of the mitral valve, the result of "dynamic" left ventricular outflow tract obstruction [9]. Physiologic cardiac adaptation secondary to regular exercise (athlete's heart) may lead to an increase in left ventricular wall thickness which may be difficult to distinguish from pathologic changes of HCM [22]. The histologic hallmark of the disease is the so called "myocardial disarray" which consists of widespread, bizzarre and disordered arrangement of myocites (Fig. 1B); the associated diffuse interstitial fibrosis is an acquired

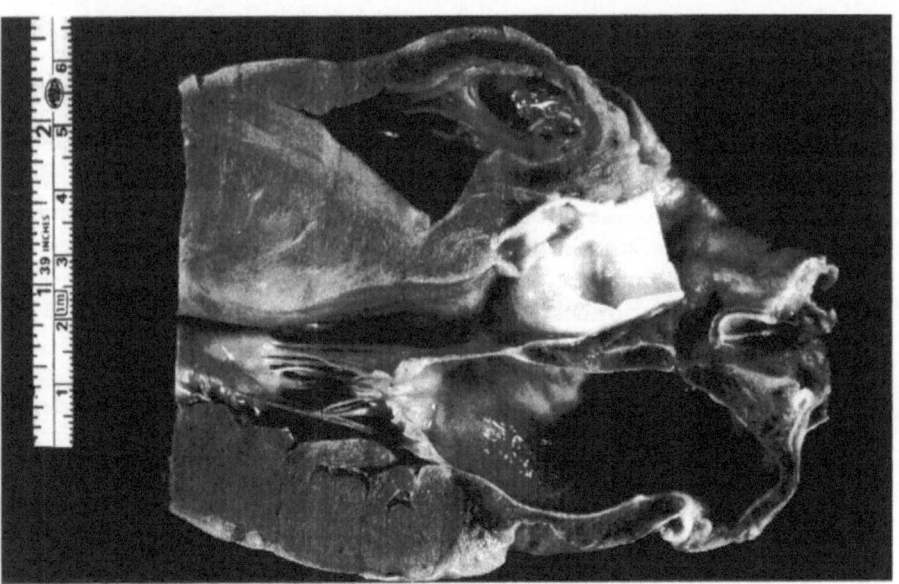

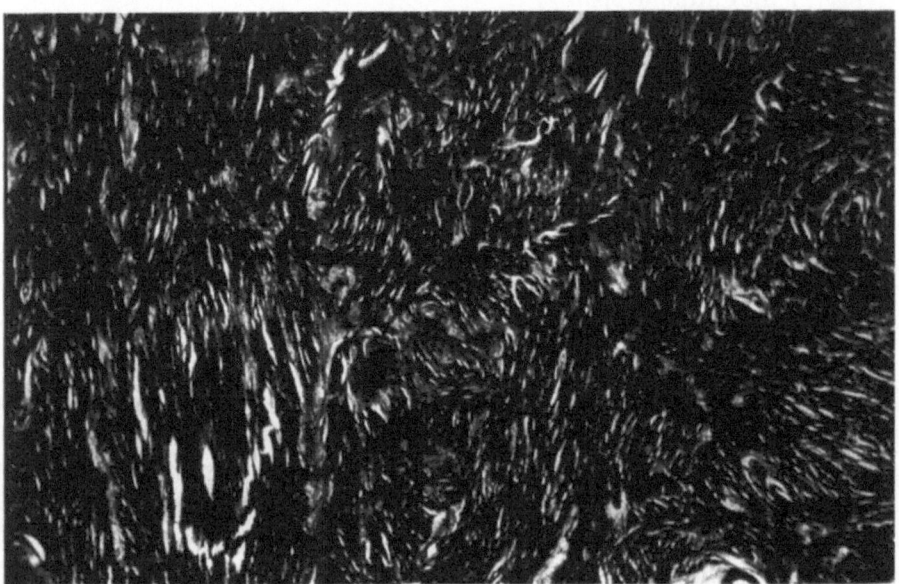

Fig. 1. Sudden death from hypertrophic cardiomyopathy in a 20-year old athlete. A) Long axis view of the heart showing "asymmetric" left ventricular hypertrophy with disproportionate septal thickening. B) At histology, architectural disarrangement of myocardial fibres ("myocardial disarray") associated with both interstitial and replacementtype fibrosis. Azan stain, original magnification x 63

phenomenon, in part related to a progressive disease of the intramural coronary arteries which show a dysplasia of the tunica media with or without lumen obstruction ("small vessel disease") [3, 6, 9]. Additional histologic signs of acute (contraction band and coagulative necrosis) and/or healed (gross septal scars and/or extensive replacement fibrosis) myocardial injury may be found in young athletes who died suddenly [23].

Sudden cardiac arrest in athletes with HCM has been attributed to primary ventricular arrhythmias [24, 25] most likely arising from the dysplastic myocardium. The observation of acquired myocardial damage, either acute or in the setting of large septal scars, supports the hypothesis that myocardial ischemia intervenes in the natural history of the disease and contributes to the arrhythmogenicity [23, 26]. Other potential mechanisms of syncope and cardiac arrest in HCM include paroxysmal supraventricular arrhythmias, AV block, and hypothension due to inappropriate vasodilator response to exercise [25, 27].

Arrhythmogenic Right Ventricular Cardiomyopathy

Arrhythmogenic right ventricular cardiomyopathy (ARVC) is a heart muscle disorder that is characterized pathologically by fibro-fatty replacement of right ventricular myocardium. The disease is often familial with an autosomal dominant pattern of inheritance and its most frequent clinical presentation consists of arrhythmias of right ventricular (RV) origin and sudden death [7, 10, 28, 29]. Since the left ventricle is usually spared, cardiac performance may be normal, thus allowing young affected subjects to face strenuous exercise. At macroscopic examination the heart of young competitive athletes dying suddenly from ARVC discloses no or only slight right ventricular dilatation and massive transmural fibro-fatty replacement of the RV muscolature (Fig. 2A) which accounts for aneurysms (infundibular, inferior, and apical), scarring fibrosis and/or large areas of very thin, translucent wall. This gross appearence of the RV allows definitive differential diagnosis from training-induced RV changes ("athlete's heart"), usually consisting in global RV enlargement [22]. Histologically, fibro-fatty atrophy of RV myocardium (Fig. 2B) is often associated with signs of focal myocardial degeneration and necrosis with patchy inflammatory infiltrates [10, 29, 30]. The fibrosis is of the replacement type and suggests a post-necrotic scarring process. The arrhythmogenicity of ARVC is reasonably explained by the widespread, irregular disruption of the RV myocardium and electrical wavefront, with inhomogeneous conduction and activation from site to site, which predisposes to the onset of malignant re-entrant ventricular tachyarrhythmias [29]

The propensity for ARVC to precipitate "arrhythmic" sudden cardiac arrest during physical exercise is most likely linked to some hemodynamic and neurohumoral factors. Physical exercise has the opposite effect on right and left ventricle and it results in acute disproportionate increase in RV afterload and cavity enlargement [32-34] which, in turn, may elicit ventricular arrhythmias by "stretching" the diseased right ventricular musculature. Progression of the

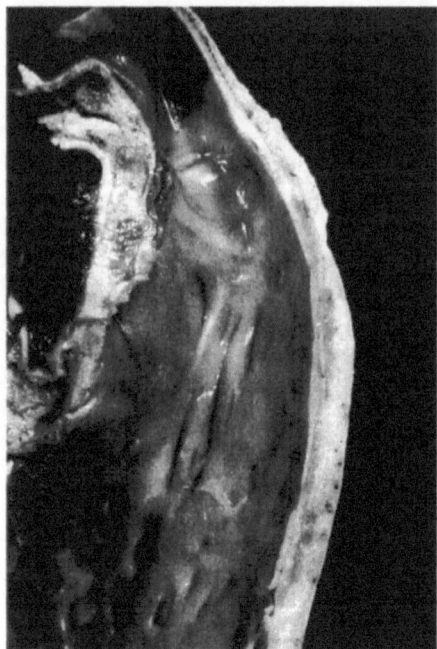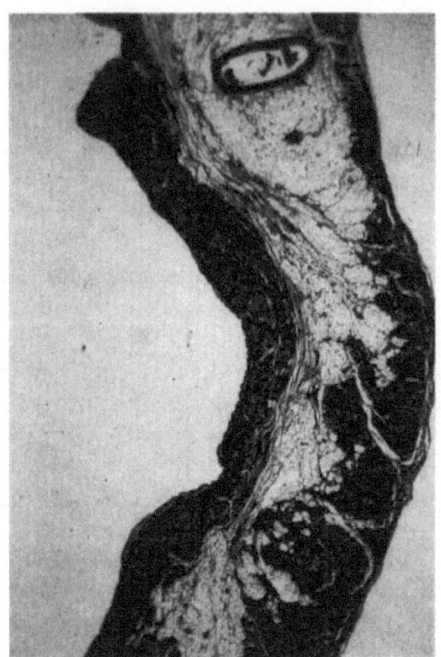

Fig. 2. Sudden death from arrhythmogenic right ventricular cardiomyopathy in a 19-year-old athlete. **A&B)** Gross and histologic feature of right ventricular outflow tract revealing remarkable fatty replacement of the ventricular myocardium. Weigert Van Gieson stain, original magnification x 6

disease from the epicardium to the endocardium might account for a functional and/or structural sympathetic denervation (sympathetic nerve trunks travel in the subepicardial layer), with supersensitivity to catecholamines and enhanced arrhythmogenicity during sympathetic stimulation [35, 36].

Early identification of ARVC plays a crucial role in the prevention of sudden fatal cardiac arrest during sport. Most athletes who died suddenly from ARVC had a history of subjective and/or objective signs of ventricular electrical instability, consisting of palpitations and/or syncopal episodes accompanying ventricular tachyarrhythmias with left bundle branch block morphology [7]. Moreover, ARVC is strongly suggested by the ECG finding of inverted T waves in right precordial leads. Definitive diagnosis is based on the echocardiographic visualization of global ventricular enlargement and/or regional right ventricular structural wall motion abnormalities [37] and, in selected cases, by magnetic resonance imaging [38] and right ventricular angiography with endomyocardial biopsy [39-41].

Congenital Coronary Anomalies

Anomalolous Coronary Artery Origin

The anomalous origin of a coronary artery from the "wrong" coronary sinus is a "minor" coronary anomaly with a silent clinical course which may precipitate sudden and unexpected ischemic cardiac arrest in young competitive athletes [6, 7, 11, 12, 42, 43]. The most frequent anatomic findings consist of both (left and right) coronary arteries arising either from the right or the left coronary sinus [42, 43]. In both conditions, as the anomalous coronary vessel leaves the aorta it shows an acute angle with the aortic wall and, thus, usually runs between the aorta and the pulmonary trunk following an early aortic intramural course, with a "slit-like" lumen [11, 12]. Pathologic examination of the ventricular myocardium usually reveals signs of acute or healed ischemic damage in the territory supplied by the anomalous coronary vessel. Fatal myocardial ischemia has been related to exercise-induced aortic root expansion which compresses the anomalous vessel against the pulmonary trunk and increases the acute angulation of the coronary take-off so aggravating the "slit-like" shape of the lumen of the proximal intramural portion of the aberrant coronary vessel [11, 12, 42, 43]. This mechanism of myocardial ischemia is difficult to reproduce in the clinical setting, as shown by the occurrence of false negative ECG exercise testing in a young athlete who subsequently died suddenly from the above coronary anomaly [11, 12].

Intramyocardial Coronary Course

Although the intramyocardial course of a coronary artery has long been regarded as a normal anatomical variant, recent clinical studies showed that this condition can lead to myocardial ischemia manifested as angina, myocardial infarction and sudden death [8, 12, 44]. Pathological studies showed ischaemic damage at various stages of healing in the myocardial territory supplied by intramural coronary arteries [12, 45]. Effort-induced ischaemia in athletes has been attributed to tachycardia which increases the myocardial oxygen requirement and reduces the coronary flow during diastole. Other proposed mechanisms include vasospasm in the intramural coronary segment and the transient formation of platelet aggregates and/or thrombosis provoked by mechanical trauma of the vessel wall. An intramural coronary artery may cause ischaemic cardiac arrest when it follows a particularly deep and long intramyocardial course [12]. The ventricular myocardium surrouding the anomalous vessel may be dysplastic and organised to form a "sheath" encircling the intramural coronary segment. This myocardial ring might cause paroxysmal obstruction of the intramural coronary vessel by inducing "extrinsic" prolonged constriction. Alternatively, the myocardial disarray and fibrosis might act as a "restrictive" perivascular tissue to limit the diastolic flow in the coronary segment, mostly during physical exercise when there is an increase of myocardial oxygen demand [12].

Other Cardiovascular Substrates

Mitral Valve Prolapse

Despite its high prevalence in the general population, mitral valve prolapse seems to be a rare cause of sudden death in athletes [7, 8]. The pathogenesis of the sudden cardiac arrest is still unknown; fatal coronary embolism from atrial platelet deposits and cardiac arrest due to malignant ventricular tachyarrhythmias attributed to "valve friction" have been advanced as possible mechanisms [46]. Sudden death has also been correlated with ventricular electrical instability due to an underlying, undiagnosed silent heart disease, such as conduction system abnormalities [47], hypertrophic cardiomyopathy [46] and right ventricular cardiomyopathy [48-50].

Conduction System Abnormalities

Congenital or acquired isolated conduction system abnormalities may represent a concealed morphologic substrate of exercise-related sudden death [7, 51]. In three young competitive athletes with apparently normal hearts on routine gross and histologic examination, the study of the conduction system by serial sections disclosed an accessory pathway in two (atrioventricular and nodoventricular respectively) and sclerocalcific interruption of the His bundle and branches in one [7]. In the absence of prodromal symptoms and ECG recordings, premortem identification of these silent conduction system abnormalities remains a challenge.

Myocarditis

Myocarditis, either in its active or healed forms, may provide a concealed myocardial electrical substate for ventricular arrhythmias and exercise-related sudden death [6, 51]. The gross appearence of the heart is not distinctive ("apparently" normal heart) while histologic examination discloses foci of mononuclear inflammatory infiltrates with areas of myocardial necrosis; concomitant areas of replacement fibrosis suggests a subacute-healed form of myocarditis. Fatal events in athletes seems unpredictable since focal myocarditis is often clinically silent and endomyocardial biopsy may fail to detect the inflammation because of sampling error.

Aortic Dissection

Spontaneous laceration of the ascending aorta with rupture into the pericardial cavity and cardiac tamponade is a rare cause of fatal "electromechanical dissociation" during sports [6, 7]. The basic heart defect is an elastic fragmentation of the aortic tunica media with cystic medial necrosis that may present rarely as an isolated histologic feature [52], but more frequently in association with isthmic coartation and/or bicuspid aortic valve [53-55], or in the setting of Marfan syndrome [56].

This study was supported by the Juvenile Sudden Death Research Project of the Veneto Region, Venice, and by the National Council for Research, Target Project FATMA, Rome, Italy.

References

1. Buddington RS, Stahl CJI, McAllister HA, et al (1974) Sports, death and unusual heart disease. Am J Cardiol 33:129
2. Thompson PD, Stern MP, Williams P, et al (1979) Death during jogging or running; a study of 18 cases. JAMA 242:1265
3. Maron BJ, Roberts WC, McAllister MA, et al (1980) Sudden death in young athletes. Circulation 62:218-29
4. Waller BF, Roberts WC (1980) Sudden death while running in conditioned runners aged 40 years or over. Am J Cardiol 45:1292
5. Virmani R, Robinowitz M, McAllister HA (1982) Nontraumatic death in joggers. Am J Med 72:874
6. Maron BJ, Epstein SE, Roberts WC (1986) Causes of sudden death in competitive athletes. J Am Coll Cardiol 7:204
7. Corrado D, Thiene G, Nava A, Pennelli N, Rossi L (1990) Sudden death in young competitive athletes: clinico-pathologic correlations in 22 cases. Am J Med 89:588-96
8. Burke AP, Farb A, Virmani R, et al (1991) Sports-related and non-sports-related sudden cardiac death in young adults. Am Heart J 121:568
9. Maron BJ, Roberts WC, Epstein SE (1982) Sudden death in hypertrophic cardiomyopathy: A profile of 78 patients. Circulation 65:1388
10. Thiene G, Nava A, Corrado D, Rossi L, Pennelli N (1988) Right ventricular cardiomyopathy and sudden death in young people. N Engl J Med 318:129
11. Virmani R, Rogan K, Cheitlin MD: Congenital coronary artery anomalies: Pathologic aspects. In Virmani R, Forman MB (eds) (1989) Nonatherosclerotic Ischemic Heart Disease. New York, Raven Press, p. 153
12. Corrado D, Thiene G, Cocco P, Frescura C (1992) Non-atherosclerotic coronary artery disease and sudden death in the young. Br Heart J 68:601-7
13. Topaz 0, Edwards JE (1985) Pathologic features of sudden death in children, adolescents, and young adults. Chest 87:476-82
14. Thiene G, Pennelli N, Rossi L (1983)Cardiac conduction system abnormalities as a possible cause of sudden death in young athletes. Hum Pathol 14:70-4
15. Noakes TD, Opie HL, Rose AG, et al (1979) Autopsy-proved coronary atherosclerosis in marathon runners. N Engl J Med 310:86
16. Ciampricotti R, El Gamal M, Relik T et al (1990) Clinical characteristics and coronary angiographic findings of patients with unstable angina, acute myocardial infarction, and survivors of sudden ischemic death occurring during or after sport. Am J Cardiol 120:1267-1278
17. Northcote RJ, Ballantyne D (1983) Sudden cardiac death in sport. Br Med J 287:1357
18. Corrado D, Thiene G, Pennelli N (1988) Sudden death as the first manifestation of coronary artery disease in young people (≤35 years). Eur Heart J 9:139-44

19. Corrado D, Basso C, Poletti A, Angelini A, Valente M, Thiene G (1994) Sudden death in the young. Is coronary thrombosis the major precipitating factor? Circulation 90:2315-323

20. Solomon SD, Jarcho JA, McKenna WJ, et al (1990) Familial hypertrophic cardiomyopathy is a genetically heterogenous disease. J Clin Invest 86:993-9

21. Thierfelder L, Watkins H, MacRae C, et al (1994) Alpha-tropomyosin and cardiac troponin Y mutations cause familial hypertrophic cardiomyopathy: a disease of the sarcomere. Cell 77:701-12

22. Maron BJ, Pelliccia A, Spirito P (1995) Cardiac disease in young trained athletes. Insights into methods for distinguishing athlete's heart from structural heart disease, with particular emphaisis on hypertrophic cardiomyopathy. Circulation 91:1596-1601

23. Basso C, Frescura C, Corrado D, et al (1995) Congenital heart disease and sudden death in theyoung. Hum Pathol 26:1065-72

24. Mc Kenna WJ, England D, Doi YL, Deanfield JE, Oakley C, Goodwin JF (1981) Arrhythmia in hypertrophic cardiomyopathy. I: influence on prognosis. Br Heart J 46: 168-72

25. Mc Kenna WJ, Camm AJ (1989) Sudden death in hypertrophic cardiomyopathy: assessment of patients at high risk.Circulation 80:1489-92

26. Dilsizian V, Bonow RO, Epstein SE, et al (1993) Myocardial ischemia detected by Thallium scintigraphy is frequently related to cardiac arrest and syncope in young patients with hypertrophic cardiomyopathy. J Am Coll Cardiol 22:796-804

27. Frenneaux MP, Counihan PJ, Caforio ALP, Chikamori T, Mc Kenna WJ (1990) Abnormal blood pressure response during exercise in hypertrophic cardiomyopathy. Circulation 82:1995-2002

28. Marcus FI, Fontaine GH, Guiraudon G, et al (1982) Right ventricular dysplasia: a report of 24 cases. Circulation 65:384-398

29. Thiene G, Corrado D, Nava A, Rossi L, Poletti A, Boffa GM, Daliento L, Pennelli N (1991) Right ventricular cardiomyopathy: is there evidence of an inflammatory etiology? Eur Heart J 12:22-5

30. Basso C, Thiene G, Corrado D, Angelini A, Nava A, Valente ML (1996) Arrhythmogenic right ventricular cardiomyopathy. Dysplasia, dystrophy, or myocarditis? Circulation 94:983-991

31. Fontaine G, Frank R, Tonet JL, et al (1984) Arrhythmogenic right ventricular dysplasia; a clinical model for the study of chronic ventricular tachycardia. Jpn Circ J48:515-38

32. Douglas PS, O'Toole ML, Hiller WDB, Reichek N (1990) Different effects of prolonged exercise on the right and left ventricles. J Am Coll Cardiol 15:64-9

33. Gurtner HP, Walser P, Fassler B (1975) Normal values for pulmonary hemodynamics at rest and during exercise in man. Prog Respir Res 9:295-315

34. Stanek V, Widirnsky J, DeBre S, Denolin H (1975) The lesser circulation during exercise in healthy subjects. Prog Respir Res 9:1-9

35. Inoue H, Zipes DP (1987) Results of sympathetic denervation in the canine heart: supersensitivity that may be arrhythmogenic. Circulation 75:877-887

36. Wichter T, Hemdricks G, Lerch H, et al (1994) Regional myocardial sympathetic dysinnervation in arrhythmogenic right ventricular cardiomyopathy. Circulation 89:667-683

37. Nava A, Thiene G, Canciani B, et al (1988) Familial occurrence of right ventricular dysplasia: a study of nine families. J Am Coll Cardiol 12:1222-8

38. Ricci C, Longo R, Pagnan L, Dalla Palma L, Pinamonti B, Camerini F, Bussani R,

Silvestri F (1992) Magnetic resonance imaging in right ventricular dysplasia. Am J Cardiol 70:1589-95

39. Blomstrom-Lundqvist C, Selin K, Jonsson R, Johansson SR, Schlossman D,Olsson SB (1988) Cardioangiographic findings in patients with arrhythmogenic right ventricular dysplasia. Br Heart J 59: 556-63

40. Daliento L, Rizzoli G, Thiene G, Nava A, Rinuncini M, Chioin R, Dalla Volta S (1990) Diagnostic accuracy of right ventricular ventriculography in arrhythmogenic right ventricular cardiomyopathy. Am J Cardiol 66:741-5

41. Angelini A, Thiene G, Boffa GM, Calliari I, Daliento L, Valente M, Chioin R, Nava A, Dalla Volta S (1993) Endomyocardial biopsy in right ventricular cardiomyopathy. Int J Cardiol 40:273-282

42. Cheitlin MD, De Castro CM, McAllister HA (1994) Sudden death as a complication of anomalous left coronary origin from the anterior sinus of Valsalva: A not so minor congenital anomaly. Circulation 50:780-7

43.   Roberts WC, Siegel RJ, Zipes DP (1982) Origin of the right coronary artery from the left sinus of Valsalva and its functional consequences: Analysis of 10 necropsy patients. Am J Cardiol 49:863-868

44. Vasan RS, Bahl VK, Rajani M (1989) Myocardial infarction associated with a myocardial bridge. Int J Cardiol 25:240-241

45. Morales AR, Romanelli R, Boucek RJ (1980) The mural left anterior descending coronary artery, strenous exercise and sudden death. Circulation 62:250-257

46. Chesler E, King RA, Edwards JE (1983) Clinicopathologic findings in sudden death attributable to the myxomatous mitral valve. Circulation 67:632-9

47. Bharati S, Granston AS, Liebson PR, et al (1981) The conduction system in mitral valve prolapse syndrome with sudden death. Am Heart J 101:667-70

48. Nava A, Thiene G (1988) Right ventricular cardiomyopathy and sudden death in young people (Letter) N Engl J Med 174: 319

49. Corrado D, Thiene G, Nava A, Rossi L (1993) Arrhythmogenic pathologic substrates of juvenile sudden death in mitral valve prolapse. J Am Coll Cardiol 21 (abstract): 242A

50. Martini B, Basso C, Thiene G (1994) Sudden death in mitral valve prolapse with Holter monitoring-documented ventricular fibrillation: evidence of coexisting arrhythmogenic right ventricular cardiomyopathy. Int J Cardiol 49:274-8

51. Corrado D, Basso C, Angelini A, Thiene G (1995) Sudden arrhythmic death in young people with apparently normal heart. Abstracts of the 44th Annual Scientific Session, American College of Cardiology. New Orleans, Louisiana. 22, J Am Coll Cardiol

52. Pachulski RT, Weinberg Al., Chan KW (1991) Aortic aneurysm in patients with functionally normal or minimally stenotic bicuspid aortic valve. Am J Cardiol 67:781-782

53. Edwards JE (1972) Aneurysms of the thoracic aorta complicating coarctation. Circulation 48:195-201

54. Edwards WD, Leaf DS, Edwards JE (1978) Dissecting aortic aneurysm associated with congenital bicuspid aortic valve. Circulation 57:1022-1025

55. Roberts CS, Roberts WC (1991) Dissection of the aorta associated with congenital malformation of aortic valve. J Am Coll Cardiol 17:712-716

56. Roberts WC, Honig HS (1982) The spectrum of cardiovascular disease in the Marfan syndrome: A clinicopathologic study of 18 necropsy patients and comparison to 151 previously reported necropsy patients. Am Heart J 104: 115-125

Methods for Distinguishing Athlete's Heart from Structural Heart Disease, with Emphasis on Hypertrophic Cardiomyopathy

B.J. Maron

Cardiovascular Research Division, Minneapolis Heart Institute Foundation, Minneapolis, Minnesota, USA

In young competitive athletes, the differential diagnosis between physiologic, nonpathologic changes in cardiac morphology associated with training (commonly referred to as "athlete's heart") [1] and certain cardiac diseases with the potential for sudden death represents an important and not uncommon clinical problem. Such crucial diagnostic distinctions often involve hypertrophic cardiomyopathy (HCM) [2], which is the most comon cause of sudden death in young competitive athletes [3].

Distinctions between athlete's heart and cardiac disease has particularly important implications, since identification of a cardiovascular abnormality in an athlete may be the basis for disqualification from competition, in an effort to minimize risk for sudden death [4]. By the same token, the improper diagnosis of cardiac disease in a normal athlete may lead to unnecessary withdrawal from athletics, thereby depriving that individual of the benefits of sport.

Differential Diagnosis Between Athlete's Heart and Cardiovascular Disease

Dilated Cardiomyopathy

In an important minority of athletes, the increase in left ventricular end-diastolic cavity dimension that occurs with training overlaps which is characteristic of certains pathologic entities. While left ventricular cavity dimension in athletes is usually in the range of 53 to 58 mm, in some individuals it may extend into what is regarded as the pathological range of > 60 mm (up to 70 mm), and thereby resemble dilated cardiomyopathy. However, the absence of left ventricular systolic dysfunction is usually sufficient to distinguish such physiologic ventricular enlargement induced by training from dilated cardiomyopathy. Nevertheless, the truly long-term consequences of marked left ventricular enlargement as part of the athlete's heart syndrome is not entirely resolved.

Arrhythmogenic Right Ventricular Dysplasia

Because highly trained athletes may demonstrated right ventricular enlargement and a variety of depolarization, repolarization, and conduction abnormalities on the ECG, the differential diagnosis between athlete's heart and arrhythmogenic right ventricular dysplasia may arise. Identification of right ventricular dysplasia by echocardiography may be exceedingly difficult, because of technical limitations in imaging right heart morphology (and assessing right ventricular function), and also because the spectrum of disease is broad [5]. Demonstration of right ventricular segmental or global dysfunction or substantial cavity enlargement supports the diagnosis. Magnetic resonance imaging however, affords a more reliable noninvasive diagnosis of this condition. The role of myocardial biopsy in the diagnosis of right ventricular dysplasia is unresolved.

Hypertrophic Cardiomyopathy

The dilemma of clinically distinguishing between athlete's heart and structural heart disease most frequently arises with respect to hypertrophic cardiomyopathy (HCM). While at present there is no single approach that will definitively resolve this question in all such athletes, several strategies are described here that alone or in combination offer a large measure of clarification in most instances for this often compelling differential diagnosis [2] (Fig. 1). The definition of HCM employed here is that of a patient (or athlete) with evidence of a hypertrophied and nondilated left ventricle in the absence of another cardiac or systemic disease that could itself produce hypertrophy of the magnitude present in that individual [6].

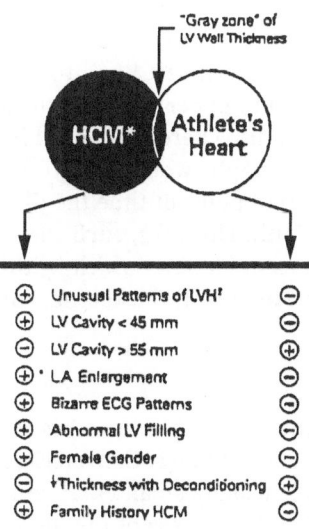

Fig. 1. Chart showing criteria used to distinguish hypertrophic cardiomyopathy (HCM) from athlete's heart when the left ventricular (LV) wall thickness is within the shaded gray zone of overlap, consistent with both diagnoses. * Assumed to be the nonobstructive form of HCM in this discussion, since the presence of substantial mitral valve systolic anterior motion would confirm, per se, the diagnosis of HCM in an athlete. † May involve a variety of abnormalities, including heterogeneous distribution of left ventricular hypertrophy (LVH) in which asymmetry is prominent, and adjacent regions may be of greatly different thicknesses, with sharp transitions evident between segments; also, patterns in which the anterior ventricular septum is spared from the hypertrophic process and the region of predominant thickening may be in the posterior portion of septum, or anterolateral or posterior free wall. ↓ = decreased; LA = left atrial
From [2]

Wall Thickness

In the vast mayority of competitive athletes, absolute left ventricular wall thickness is within normal limits(≤12 mm). In some athletes, however, left ventricular wall thickness may be more substantial, 13-15 mm, unavoidably raising the possibility of HCM [7]. In patients with HCM, the increase in left ventricular wall thickness is usually marked; the average wall thickness reported in most echocardiographic studies of this disease is ≈20 mm, and ranging up to 60 mm [8, 9]. However, an important minority of patients with HCM show relatively mild left ventricular hypertrophy with wall thickness values in the range of ≈13 to 15 mm, and most of these patients are asymptomatic. Therefore, a diagnostic dilemma may arise in those athletes who fall into this morphological "gray zone" between physiological hypertrophy and HCM with maximal wall thickness of 13 or 14 mm, or possibly 15 mm [2].

In highly trained athletes, the region of predominant left ventricular wall thickening always involves the anterior septum, although the thicknesses of other segments of the wall are similar (with differences in the range of 1 to 2 mm). In patients with HCM, the anterior portion of the ventricular septum is also usually the region of maximal wall thickening; however, the pattern of hypertrophy is often heterogeneous, asymmetry is prominent, and occasionally regions other than the anterior septum may show the most marked thickening [8, 9]. In addition, contiguous portions of the left ventricle often show strikingly different wall thicknesses in HCM, and the treansition between such areas is often sharp and abrupt [8, 9].

Diagnosis of HCM in asymptomatic athletes is frequently based solely on echocardiographic assessment of the magnitude of hypertrophy, and often of precise quantitative mausurements of wall thickness in a single segment or region of the left ventricular wall. It should be emphasized that, in borderline cases, such circumstances present fertile ground for the overdiagnosis of this disease.

Since a marked increase in left ventricular wall thickness often occurs during adolescence in patients with HCM, young athletes with HCM (< 16 years old) may not demonstrate their maximum expression of hypertrophy until full physical maturation and development is achieved [10]. Therefore, an athlete with HCM may initially be evaluated with echocardiography when hypertrophy is still only mild or within the borderline range; at that point in time the differential diagnosis with athlete's heart may be difficult. However, such uncertainty can be resolved by serial echocardiographic examinations which, within months or years, may show more definite left ventricular wall thickening, confirming the diagnosis of HCM.

Cavity Dimension

An enlarged left ventricular end-diastolic cavity dimension (> 55 mm) is present in more than one third of highly trained elite male athletes. Conversely, in patients with HCM, the diastolic cavity dimension is usually small (< 45 mm), and is > 55 mm only in those who evolve to the end-stage phase of the disease with progressive heart failure and systolic dysfunction. Therefore, in some instances, it is possible to distinguish the athlete's heart from HCM solely on the basis of left ventricular cavity dimension. However, in those athletes in whom left ventricular cavity size falls between the extremes, this dimension alone will not resolve the differential diagnosis.

ECG
Because of the wide variety of ECG alterations present in athletes without cardiovascular disease and in patients with HCM, the 12-lead ECG is not particularly usefull in distiguishing between these two entities. However, unusual and bizarre ECG patterns with strikingly increased voltages, prominent Q waves, or deep negative T waves are probably more characteristic of HCM.

Doppler Transmitral Waveform
Abnormalities of left ventricular diastolic filling have been identified noninvasively with pulsed Doppler echocardiography or radionuclide angiography in many patients with a variety of cardiac diseases associated with left ventricular hypertrophy. Most patients with HCM, including those with relatively mild hypertrophy (i.e., that could be confused with athlete's heart), show abnormal Doppler indexes of left ventricular filling independent of whether symptoms or outflow obstruction are present. Typically, the early peak of transmitral flow-velocity ("E" due to rapid filling) is decreased and deceleration time of the early peak is prolonged; the late peak ("A" due to atrial contraction) is increased, inverting the normal E/A ratio. On the other hand, trained athletes invariably demonstrate normal left ventricular filling pattern. Consequently, in a trained athlete suspected of having HCM, a distinctly abnormal Doppler transmitral flow-velocity pattern strongly supports this diagnosis, while a normal Doppler pattern is compatible with either HCM or athlete's heart [11].

Ultrasonic Myocardial Reflectively (Integrated Backscatter Signal)
Initial observations suggest that most asymptomatic (or mildly symptomatic) patients with HCM show increased intensity of the ultrasound signal from the septum and posterior free wall (including patients with mild and localized hypertrophy) while highly trained athletes with physiological hypertrophy show normal myocardial tissue reflectivity [12]. However, it is not known at present whether differences in the backscatter signal identified by group comparisons can be used to distinguish athlete's heart from cardiac disease in individual subjects.

Type of Sport Training
The specific nature of athletic training itself has a major influence on the type and magnitude of the changes in left ventricular dimensions [7, 13]. For example, in a study of almost 1000 elite Italian athletes, only about 2% had a left ventricular wall thickness a $\geq$ 13 mm (in the gray zone between physiological hypertrophy and HCM), and this subset was confined to those in rowing sports

and cycling. Conversely, most other forms of training, including isometric (or power) sports such as weight-lifting or wrestling, were not associated with absolute increases in thickness beyond 12 mm [14]. Therefore, in assessing whether or not an athlete with increased wall thickness has HCM, detailed knowledge of the training regimen is relevant. It is also possible that the outer limits of left ventricular wall thickness differ in trained athletes of various ethnic and racial origins, although this issue has not yet been fully resolved.

Gender
Gender differences with regard to alterations in cardiac dimensions and left ventricular mass have been indentified in trained athletes. Preliminary findings indicate that highly trained female athletes rarely show left ventricular wall thicknesses that are within the aforementioned gray-zone between athlete's heart and HCM. For example, in a recent report, none of 600 elite women athletes had left ventricular wall thickness in the range compatible with the diagnosis of HCM(≥13 mm) [15]. These observations suggest, therefore, that female athletics with "borderline" left ventricular wall thicknesses of 13-15 mm (in the presence of normal cavity size) are likely to have HCM.

Regression of Left Ventricular Hypertrophy with Deconditioning
The observation that increased left ventricular cavity size or wall thickness are physiological consequences of atlhetic training may be substantiated by serial echocardiographic examinations showing a decrease in cardiac dimensions and mass with deconditioning [16, 17]. Decrease in left ventricular wall thickness associated with deconditioning is inconsistent with pathologic forms of hypertrophy (i.e., HCM). The identification of such changes in wall thickness with deconditioning requires: [1] compliance from highly motivated competitive athletes to interrupt their training; and [2] serial echocardiographic studies of optimal technical quality.

Familial Transmission and Genetics
The most definitive evidence from the presence of HCM in an athlete with an increase in wall thickness probably comes from the demonstration of HCM in a relative [18]. Therefore, in those athletes in whom the distinction between HCM and athlete's heart cannot otherwise be achieved definitively, echocardiographic screening for affected family members represent a potential method for resolving this diagnostic uncertainty. The absence of HCM in family members, however, does not exclude this disease since in may be "sporadic" (i.e., absent in relatives other than the index case).

Recent advances in defining the genetic alterations responsible for HCM raise the possibility of DNA diagnosis in athletes suspected of having this disease. The genetic abnormalities that cause HCM, however, are greatly heterogeneous [19-21]. At present, mutations responsible for HCM have been identified in four genes located on chromosomes 1, 11, 14 and 15 encoding for proteins of the sarcomere - i.e., cardiac troponin T, myosin binding protein C, b-myosin heavy chain and a-tropomyosin. This substatial genetic heterogeneity has made it extremely difficult and time consuming to use techniques of molecular biology for the purpose sof clinically resolving the differential diagnosis between athlete's heart and HCM.

References

1. Maron BJ (1986) Structural features of the athlete heart as defined by echocardiography. J Am Coll Cardiol 7:190-203
2. Maron BJ, Pelliccia A, Spirito P (1995) Cardiac disease in young trained athletes: Methods for distinguishing athlete's heart from structural heart disease with particular emphasis on hypertrophic cardiomyopathy. Circulation 92:1596-1601
3. Maron BJ, Shirani J, Poliac LC, Mathenge R, Roberts WC, Mueller FO (1996) Sudden death in young competitive athletes: Clinical, dermographic and pathological profiles. JAMA 276:199-204
4. Maron BJ, Mitchell JH (1994) 26th Bethesda Conference. Recommendations for determining eligibility for competition in athletes with cardiovascular abnormalities. J Am Coll Cardiol 24:845-899
5. McKenna WJ, Thiene G, Nava A, Fontaliran F, Blomstrom-Lundqvist C, Fontaine G, Camerini F (1994) Diagnosis of arrhythmogenic right ventricular dysplasia/cardiomyopathy. Br Heart J 71:215-218
6. Maron BJ, Epstein SE (1979) Hypertrophic cardiomyopathy: A discussion of nomenclature. Am J Cardiol 43:1242-1244
7. Pelliccia A, Maron BJ, Spataro A, Proschan MA, Spirito P (1991) The upper limit of physiologic cardiac hypertophy in highly trained elite athletles. N Engl J Med 324:295-301
8. Maron BJ, Gottdiener JS, Epstein SE (1981) Patterns and significance of the distribution of left ventricular hypertrophy in hypertrophic cardiomyopathy: A wide-angle, two-dimensional echocardiographic study of 125 patients. Am J Cardiol 48:418-428
9. Klues HG, Schiffers A, Maron BJ (1995) Phenotypic spectrum and petterns of left ventricular hypertrophy in hypertrophic cardiomyopathy: Morphologic observation and significance as assessed by two-dimensional echocardiography in 600 patients. J Am Coll Cardiol 26:1699-1708
10. Maron BJ, Spirito P, Wesley Y, Arce J (1985) Development and progression of left ventricular hypertrophy in children with hypertrophic cardiomyopathy. N Engl J Med 315:610-614
11. Lewis JF, Spirito P, Pelliccia A, Maron BJ (1992) Usefulness of Doppler echocardiographic assessment of diastolic filling in distinguishing "athlete's heart" from hypertrophic cardiomyopathy. Br Heart J 68:296-300
12. Lattanzi F, Spirito P, Picano E, Mazzarisi A, Landini L, Distante A, Vecchio C, L'Abbate A (1991) Quantitative assessment of ultrasonic myocardial reflectivity in hypertrophic cardiomyopathy. J Am Coll Cardiol 17:1085-1090
13. Spirito P, Pelliccia A, Proschan MA, Granata M, Spataro A, Caselli G, Biffi A, Vecchio C, Maron BJ (1994) Morphology of the "athlete's heart" assessed by echocardiography in 947 elite athletes representing 27 sports. Am J Cardiol 74:802-806
14. Pelliccia A, Maron BJ, Spataro A, Caselli G (1993) Absence of left ventricular hypertrophy in athletes engaged in intense power training. Am J Cardiol 72:1048-1054
15. Pelliccia A, Maron BJ, Culasso F, Spataro A, Caselli G (1996) Athlete's heart in

women: Echocardiographic characterization of highly trained elite female athletes. JAMA 276:211-215

16. Maron BJ, Pelliccia A, Spataro A, Granata M (1993) Reduction in left ventricular wall thickness after deconditioning in highly trained Olympic athletes. Br Heart J 69:125-128

17. Ehsani AA, Hagberg JM, Hickson RC (1978) Rapid changes in left ventricular dimension and mass in response to physical conditioning and deconditioning. Am J Cardiol 42:52-26

18. Maron BJ, Nichols PF, Pickle LW, Wesley YE, Mulvihill JJ (1984) Patterns of inheritance in hypertrophic cardiomyopathy: Assessment by M-mode and two-dimensional echocardiography. Am J Cardiol 53:1087-1094

19. Thierfelder L, Watkins H, MacRae C, Lamas R, McKenna WJ, Vosberg HP, Seidman JG, Seidman CE (1994) a-Tropomyosin and cardiac troponin T mutations cause familial hypertrophic cardiomyopathy: A disease of the sarcomere. Cell 77:701-712

20. Watkins H, Rosenzweig A, Hwang DS, Levi T, McKenna UJ, Seidman CE, Seidman JG (1992) Characteristics and prognostic implications of myosin missense mutations in familial hypertrophic cardiomyopathy. N Engl J Med 326:1108-1114

21. Watkins H, Conner D, Thierfelder L, Jarcho JA, Suk HJ, McRae C, McKenna WJ, Maron BJ, Seidman JG, Seidman CE (1995) Mutations in the cardiac myosin binding protein-C gene on chromosome 11 cause familial hypertrophic cardiomyopathy. Nature Genetics 11:434-437

Sudden Cardiac Death in Competitive Athletes

B.J. Maron

Cardiovascular Research Division, Minneapolis Heart Institute Foundation, Minneapolis, Minnesota, USA

Over the past 15-20 years there has been heightened awareness that highly trained young individuals participating in competitive sporting activities may harbor underlying structural cardiovascular disease [1]. The fact that many such athletes may have partecipated at exceptionally high levels of excellence for long period of time with severe cardiovascular malformations has intrigued investigators and the lay public [1]. Recognition that athletic field catastrophes may be due to a variety of detectable cardiovascular lesions has also stimulated intense interest in preparticipation screening [2-5], as well as issues related to criteria for disqualification and eligibility [6].

Sudden death in young athletes is usually instantaneous and occurs predomintly on the athletic field during competition or training; at present, the vast majority of these deaths are in men. Uncommonly, premonitory symptoms are evident and very rarely is the correct cardiovascular diagnosis made during life. Indeed, the standard preparticipation history and physical examination almost uniformly fails to indentify cardiovascular disease in those competitive athletes who ultimately die; only occasionally is a specific diagnosis made or suspected.

Over the last several years there have been a number of surveys designed to define the frequency with which a variety of cardiovascular lesions cause sudden death in different athletic populations [7-12]. Each of these studies is subject to a certain degree of patient selection bias, due largely to the lack of a systemmatic registry available for prospective identification and tabulation of athletic field deaths. Most of these analyses have focused on the youthfull athlete. Furthermore, the majority of these date sets incriminate a broad spectrum of diseases, encompassing virtually all lesions known to cause sudden death in young individuals (whether or not they are athletes) (Table 1).

The diseases responsible for sudden death do not occur with the same frequency. The most common single cardiovascular abnormality among these would appear to be hypertrophic cardiomyopathy (HCM), usually in the nonobstructive form [13]. The prevalence of HCM in such study populations is in the range of 33% [10]. Indeed, in hospital and outpatient-based patient series, HCM has proved to have a predilection for young and asymptomatic individuals, similar to athletic populations.

Table 1. Cardiovascular abnormalities in 134 young competitive athletes with sudden death

Primary Cardiovascular Lesions	No. (%) of Athletes	Median Age (Range), years
Hypertrophic cardiomyopathy	48 (36.0)	17.0 (13-28)
Unexplained increase in cardiac mass† ("possible hypertrophic cardiomyopathy")	14 (10.0)	15.0 (14-24)
Aberrant coronary arteries‡	17 (13.0)	15.0 (12-23)
Other coronary anomalies	8 (6.0)	17.5 (14-40)
Ruptured aortic aneurysm§	6 (5.0)	17.0 (16-31)
Tunneled LAD* coronary artery	6 (5.0)	17.5 (14-20)
Aortic valve stenosis	5 (4.0)	14.0 (14-17)
Lesion consistent with myocarditis	4 (3.0)	15.5 (13-16)
Idiopathic dilated cardiomyopathy	4 (3.0)	18.0 (18-21)
ARVD*	4 (3.0)	16.0 (15-17)
Idiopathic myocardial scarring	4 (3.0)	20.0 (14-27)
Mitral valve prolapse§	3 (2.0)	16.0 (15-23)
Atherosclerotic coronary artery disease	3 (2.0)	19.0 (14-28)
Other congenital heart diseases||	2 (1.5)	13.5 (12-15)
Long QT syndrome¶	1 (0.5)	...
Sarcoidosis	1 (0.5)	...
Sickle cell trait#	1 (0.5)	...
"Normal" heart**	3 (2.0)	18.0 (16-21)

*LAD, left anterior descending; ARVD, arrhythmogenic right ventricular dysplasia
† Includes 1 athlete with grossly normal heart but distinctly abnormal histologic architecture with marked disorganization of cardiac muscle cells and bundles; also, 2 of the 13 atheltes with mildly increased mass had associated tunneled LAD coronary artery.
‡ Anomalous origin of left main coronary artery from right sinus of Valsalva in 13, anomalous origin of the right coronary artery from left sinus of Valsalva in 2, anomalous origin of the left main (from between the left and posterior cusps) with acute-angled take-off in 1, and origin of LAD coronary artery from pulmonary trunk in 1.
§ Marfan syndrome was also present in 3 athletes with ruptured aortic aneurysm and in 1 with mitral valve prolapse.
|| One athlete with secundum atrial septal defect and 1 with coarctation of aorta.
¶ Also had anomalous origin of right coronary artery from left sinus of Valsalva.
# Judged to be the probable cause of death in the absence of any identifiable structure cardiovascular abnormality.
** Absence of structural heart disease on standard autopsy examination.

While HCM may be suspected during preparticipation sports evaluations by the prior occurence of exertional syncope, family history of the disease or premature cardiac death, or by a loud heart murmur, such features are relatively uncommon among all individuals affected by this disease. In addition, we not infrequently encounter at autopsy hearts with increased mass (and wall thichness) and non-dilated left ventricular cavity suggestive of HCM, but in which the objective morphologic findings are not sufficiently striking to permit a definitive diagnosis of HCM. It is uncertain whether some of these cases (often referred to as idiopathic left ventricular hypertrophy) represent mild morphologic expressions of HCM [14], unusual instances of "athlete's heart" [15] with non-benign consequences, or possibly examples of undetected right ventricular dysplasia with left ventricular hypertrophy.

Second in importance and frequency to HCM is a spectrum of congenital vascular malformations of the coronary arterial tree (in about 20%), the most common of which appears to be anomalous origin of the left main coronary artery from the right sinus of Valsalva [16]. This lesion is of particular clinical inportance, since it is rarely identified during life, but nevertheless is theoretically amenable to corrective surgery. Coronary artery anomalies are difficult to identify in patients because they are not often readily identifiable by conventional noninvasive imaging technology or simply because the clinical index of suspicion has not been sufficiently high. Such patients may die suddenly as the first manifestation of their disease, or alternatively experience one or more episodes of syncope - presumably on the basis of acute myocardial ischemia caused by the anatomic bend taken by the anomalous left main coronary artery. Other coronary anomalies apparently responsible for youthfull athletic field deaths include anomalous origin of the right coronary artery (the anatomic mirror image of anomalous left main coronary), coronary arterial hypoplasia, and occasionally premature atherosclerotic coronary artery disease.

A variety of other lesions occur as causes of sudden death in previously asymptomatic and competitive athletes with lesser (or relatively low) frequency. These include Marfan's syndrome, myocarditis, dilated cardiomyopathy, aortic valve stenosis, mitral valve prolapse, sarcoidosis, and arrhythmogenic right ventricular dysplasia. In some instances, athletes with sudden death demonstrate combined lesions - e.g. HCM associated with a coronary anomaly, or HCM with evidence of myocarditis.

In our experience, in about 2% of cases, the standard medical examiner autopsy examination fails to show a cardiovascular lesion that could account for sudden death. It is possible that death in these athletes with a "normal" autopsy is due to other conditions such as long QT syndrome (which is not associated with structural cardiac abnormalities), drug abuse (such as with cocaine), occult structural abnormalities of the conduction system, or possibly undetected examples of right ventricular dysplasia.

Certain issues related to arrhythmogenic right ventricular dysplasia [17-19] as a cause of sudden death in athletes are presently unresolved. As noted, studies from North American centers have focused on HCM and coronary anomalies as causes of sudden death in young athletes. Of great interest, however, reports from investigators from the northeastern (Veneto) region of Italy suggest a much different experience in which arrhythmogenic right ventricular dysplasia has emerged as the predominant cardiac disease encountered as an explanation for sudden death in young trained athletes [9, 18]. While this disease is also a component of our own experience with athletic field deaths, its frequency is clearly in the range of < 5% in North American reports. The explanation for such discrepancies is uncertain, although it is possible that the relatively frequent occurence of right ventricular dysplasia in a particular region of Italy reflects a unique genetic substrate. Furthermore, the relatively low frequency with which HCM is apparently responsible for sudden death in Italian athletes is an interesting but also a largely unresolved issue. It is possible that the longstanding and systematic Italian national program for the cardiovascular assessment of competitive athletes [4] has had the effect of identifying and disqualifying disproportionate numbers of trained athletes with HCM.

In addition to the risk for sudden death in athletes due to underlying and usually unsuspected cardiovascular disease, we have recently identified another mechanism for sudden catastrophe and cardiac arrest on the athletic field, but in individuals free of cardiac disease [20]. In such young athletes, blunt chest inpact over the heart produced either by a missile (such as a baseball) or by collision with another athlete (Figure 1) may induce a lethal cardiac arrhythmia and instantaneous collapse. The mechanism responsible for cardiac arrest may be as follows: induction of a premature ventricular contraction results from the chest impact which in turn induces repetitive and particularly letal ventricular arrhythmia by virtue of a R on T phenomenon - i.e., the premature beath interferes with repolarization by contacting the upstroke or peak of the T wave. Most of these occurrences have proven fatal, but a small number of survivors have now been identified, supporting the need for early recognition of the syndrome and prompt institution of cardiopulmonary resuscitation.

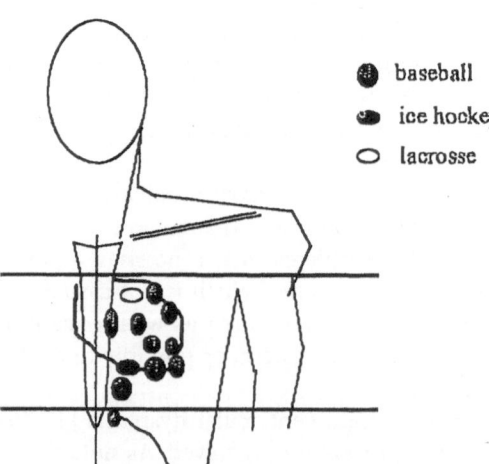

● baseball

● ice hockey

○ lacrosse

Fig. 1. Schematic representation of the location of impact points (contusions) judged to have been produced by baseballs (N=10), a hockey puck, and a lacrosse ball on the anterior chest walls of 12 victims of commotio cordis. The estimated contour of the heart is indicated by the heavy line.
(Reproduced from Maron et al. [20] with permission for the New England Journal of Medicine)

References

1. Maron BJ (1993) Sudden death in young athletes: Lessons from the Hank Gathers affair. N Engl J Med 329:55-57
2. Maron BJ, Bodison S, Wesley Y, Tucker E, Green KJ (1987) Results of screening a large population of intercollegiate athletes for cardiovascular disease. J Am Coll Cardiol 10:1214-1222
3. Lewis JF, Maron BJ, Diggs JA, Spencer JE, Mehrotra PP, Curry CL (1989) Preparticipation echocardiographic screening of cardiovascular disease in a large, predominantly black population of collegiate athletes. Am J Cardiol 64:1029-1033
4. Pelliccia A, Maron BJ (1995) Preparticipation cardiovascular evaluation of the competitive athlete: Perspectives from the 30 year Italian experience. Am J Cardiol 75:827-828
5. Maron BJ, Thompson PD, Puffer JC, McGrew CA, Strong WB, Douglas PS, Clark LT, Mitten MJ, Crawford MH, Atkins DL, Driscol DJ, Epstein AE (1996) Cardiovascular preparticipation screening of competitive athletes. A statement for health professionsl from the Sudden Death Committee (Clinical Cardiology) and Congenital Cardiac Defects Committee (Cardiovascular Disease in the Young), American Heart Association. Circulation 94:850-856
6. Maron BJ, Mitchell JH (1994) 26th Bethesda Conference. Recommendations for determining eligibility for competition in athletes with cardiovascular abnormalities. J Am Coll Cardiol 24:845-899
7. Maron BJ, Roberts WC, McAllister HA, Rosing DR, Epstein SE (1980) Sudden death in young athletes. Circulation 62:218-229
8. Burke AP, Farb A, Virmani R, Goodin J, Smialek JE (1991) Sports-related and non-sports-related sudden cardiac death in young athletes. Am Heart J 121:568-575
9. Corrado D, Thiene G, Nava A, Rossi L, Pennelli N (1990) Sudden death in young competitive athletes: Clinicopathologica correlations in 22 cases. Am J Med 39:588-596
10. Maron BJ, Shirani J, Poliac LC, Mathenge R, Roberts WC, Mueller FO (1996) Sudden death in young competitive athletes: Clinical, dermographic and pathological profiles. JAMA 276:199-204
11. Maron BJ, Epstein SE, Roberts WC (1986) Causes of sudden death in the competitive athletes. J Am Coll Cardiol 7:204-214
12. Van Camp SP, Bloor CM, Mueller FO, Cantu RC, Olson HG (1995) Nontraumatic sports death in high school and college athletes. Med Sci Sports Exer 27:641-647
13. Maron BJ, Bonow RO, Cannon RO, Leon MB, Epstein SE (1987) Hypertrophic cardiomyopathy: Interrelation of clinical manifestations, pathophysiology, and therapy. N Engl J Med 316:780-789 and 844-852
14. Spririto P, Maron BJ, Bonow RO, Epstein SE (1986) Severe functional limitation in patients with hypertrophic cardiomyopathy and only mild localized left ventricular hypertrophy. J Am Coll Cardiol 8:537-544
15. Maron BJ (1986) Structural features of the athlete heart as defined by echocardiography. J Am Coll Cardiol 7:190-203
16. Cheitlin MD, De Castro CM, McAllister HA (1974) Sudden death as a complication of anomalous left coronary origin from the anterior sinus of Valsalva, a not-so-minor congenital anomaly. Circulation 50:780-787
17. Marcus FI, Fontaine GH, Cuiraudon G, Frank R, Laurenceau JL, Malergue C, Grosgogeat Y (1982) Rigth ventricular dysplasia: A report of 24 adult cases. Circulation 65:384-398

18. Thiene G, Nava A, Corrado D, Rossi L, Penelli N (1988) Right ventricular cardiomyopathy and sudden death in young people. N Engl J Med 318:129-133
19. McKenna WJ, Thiene G, Nava A, Fontaliran F, Blomstrom-Lundqvist C, Fontaine G, Camerini F (1994) Diagnosis of arrhythmogenic right ventricular dysplasia/cardiomyopathy. Br Heart J 71:215-218
20. Maron BJ, Poliac L, Kaplan JA, Mueller FO (1995) Blunt impact to the chest leading to sudden death from cardiac arrest during sports activities. N Engl J Med 333:337-342

Physical Exercise and Ischemic Heart Disease

V. Masini

Professor Hemeritus of Cardiology Rome, Italy

The topic "Physical Exercise and Ischemic Heart Disease" can be broken down into two separate issues: 1) physical exercise as the primary form of effective prevention of ischemic heart disease and 2) the choices, limitations and benefits of physical exercise for a patient already suffering from ischemic heart disease.

This paper will focus on the second issue which is of great interest due to the considerable number of young people affected by ischemic heart disease and to the widespread desire to do sports.

The first question to ask in regard to this issue is which clinical forms of ischemic heart disease allow for physical exercise and which do not.

In order to answer this fundamental question, some information is necessary in regard to: 1) the nosography and clinical severity of ischemic heart disease; 2) the cardiovascular and metabolic effects of the various types of sports.

Nosography and Severity of Ischemic Heart Disease

The clinical manifestations of ischemic heart disease differ considerably in terms of symptoms and severity and include: stable angina, unstable angina, intermediate syndrome, myocardial infarction, chronic ischemic myocardiopathy, X syndrome, sudden death (see below). In addition, particular clinical pictures are: ischemic heart disease following revascularization procedures and post-thrombolysis myocardial infarction.

1) Stress angina is defined as stable 4 weeks after its onset: it is characterized by stress-induced anginal pain with stabilized tolerance. The course of this type of angina is generally chronic and is the result of coronary failure caused by the severe stenosis (> 70%) of one or more coronary branches.

2) All other forms of angina are defined as unstable and include: early stress angina, increased stress angina, angina at rest, post-infarction angina, Prinzmetal's vasospastic angina.

Angina at rest and post-infarction angina are the most severe. They are characterized by spontaneous anginal pain often associated with prolonged ischemic alterations. The pathogenesis of these conditions is connected with coronary failure for complicated plates associated with vasospastic phenomena. These forms of angina can evolve in various ways, for example: and change to an asymptomatic phase or stable angina, or resulting in myocardial infarction or sudden death.

3) In some cases, prolonged coronary failure causes myocardial damage not of the necrotic type but associated with prolonged electrocardiography and echocardiographic alterations, yet not involving enzymatic changes. These cases are defined "intermediate syndrome", they are linked with the same anatomical-functional coronary aspects of unstable angina and can result in functional recovery or, as is more often the case, in myocardial infarction.

4) Myocardial infarction is caused by prolonged coronary failure due to thrombotic occlusion on a complicated plate. It can either be a Q infarction or non-Q infarction depending on its extensiveness. Myocardial infarction has an early mortality of 25%, operally due to arhytmia, and a late in hospital mortality of 8%. The evolution of the infarction can be: recovery to an asymptomatic state, development of stable or unstable angina, or evolution towards a chronic dilated myocardiopathy.

5) Post-infarction myocardial damage or damage caused by prolonged angina can result in left ventricle dilation accompanied by extensive hypokinesis through a progressive process known as "ventricular remodelling": these cases are defined as chronic ischemic miocardiopathy. Such a process can be asymptomatic in the early stages but may subsequently result in heart failure or severe arrhythmia, often associated with overt or silent coronary failure. The severity of the post-ischemic dilated myocardiopathy depends on the extent of the contractile damage and the resistance to therapy. Conditions involving chronic decompensation and conditions presenting tachycardia or ventricular fibrillation are more severe.

6) The last condition, characterized by stenocardial pain, is "angina with normal coronary arteries", called X syndrome on account of its obscure aspects.

This condition is characterized by reproducible stress-induced stenocardial pain accompanied by electrocardiographic alterations in patients who do not display significant stenosis or vasospastic phenomena involving the coronary epicardial vessels. By definition, hypertension or diabetes must not be present in these cases.

X syndrome offers remarkable resistance to antiangina treatment, but has an excellent quo ad vitam prognosis as it does not lead to infarction or sudden death. The pathogenesis remains unclear although, at least in some cases, there is probably vasospastic component involving the arterioles (microvascular angina).

7) Sudden death represents the most severe form of ischemic heart disease. It can be the first and only manifestation of the disease or can complicate the course of other clinical conditions. Its pathogenesis is often arrhythmic, generally due to hyperkinetic ventricular arrhythmias (tachycardia or ventricular fibrillation) and less frequently due to hypokinetic arrhyhtmias or electromechanical dissociation.

In fortunate cases it is possible to interrupt the fatal outcome through cardiopulmonary resuscitation procedures and interruption of the arrhythmia by defibrillation; in order to do this, however, the patient must be rushed to an emergency unit within 4 minutes of cardiocirculatory arrest.

8) The natural course of ischemic heart disease can be modified considerably by medical treatment, and even more so by revascularization processes such as angioplasty or by-pass. In these patients the prognosis depends upon the success of the operation, previous myocardial damage, residual coronary failure and the potential for evolution of the coronary lesions.

Indications and Contra-indications for Physical Exercise in Subjects Suffering from Ischemic Heart Disease

The following clinical manifestations of ischemic heart disease, are considered contra-indications for sports activity: 1) early stress angina; 2) stable stress-induced angina with low tolerance (< 100 watts or a D.P. < 20,000); 3) unstable angina in the "hot phase"; 4) intermediate syndrome and infarction in the acute phase (< 2 months); 5) chronic ischemic myocardiopathy in the symptomatic stage; 6) subjects resuscitated from sudden death; 7) patients operated for revascularization with symptoms of heart failure, severe arrhythmias or coronary failure at rest or under stress with low tolerance.

The best indications for physical exercise and sports practice in the presence of ischemic heart disease are: 1) stable stress-induced angina without high tolerance (> 100 watt); 2) subjects with or without symptoms of stress angina with high tolerance following unstable angina; 3) myocardial infarction without complications; 4) early asymptomatic ischemic myocardiopathy cases; 5) asymptomatic cases after good revascularization; 6) probably the X syndrome.

Beneficial Effects of Sports Practice in Ischemic Heart Disease

Through what mechanisms can sports practice show beneficial effects in subjects suffering from ischemic heart disease?

Analyzing the various types of sports practiced, it is possible to distinguish between sports based on endurance and sports based on strength; the former determine circulatory modifications in relation to volume overloads, whereas the latter do so in relation to increases in pressure. It seems obvious that only endurance sports can be useful as for as ischemic heart disease is concerned; indeed, they generate positive hemodynamic and respiratory effects such as: a) brachycardia and higher oxygen intake with better exercise tolerance; b) vagotonia with a reduced proclivity in arrhythmia; c) metabolic effects which correct coronary risk factors like obesity, physical inactivity, overeating and dyslipidemias.

The latter effect was recently extensively investigated. It has been proven fact that physical activity increases the muscle's use of free fatty acids, supplied in part by endocellular fats or by hydrolysis of circulating lipoproteins. In the plasma there is a decrease in triglycerides and LDLs and an increase in HDL 2s that are rich in cholesterol. These effects, however, are influenced by aerobic physical activity only (3 sessions a week and demanding enough as to entail a metabolic expenditure of at least 1000 calories a week).

In addition to these advantages, it is also worth mentioning the beneficial psychological effects and the improvement in the level of post-infarction ventricular remodelling, as proven by recent Italian research studies showing a less altered ventricular diastolic diameter in infarctions treated with physical activity.

In conclusion, post-infarction rehabilitation through physical activity improves quality of life by increasing exercise tolerance, facilitating the patient's return to work and encouraging the modification of risk factors. Whether or not it determines an increase in survival and a reduction in re-infarction is as yet unknown.

Some fifteen years ago Vecchio and La Rovere (1982) compared 139 rehabilitated subjects with infarction with non-rehabilitated patients and observed a higher survival rate among the rehabilitated subjects; this study, however, was not randomized. In 1989 Harward Medical School, in collaboration with Hannover, Betheseda and Stanford Universities, undertook a major metanalysis consisting of 22 controlled and randomized studies involving a total of 2310 patients and 2244 controls who had survived myocardial infarction 15 days to 3 years earlier. The subjects were almost all males aged between 60 and 70. The treatment was physical activity, either alone or associated with pharmacological treatment. The end points were total and cardiovascular mortality, sudden death, fatal and non-fatal re-infarction. The subjects under treatment registered the following: a reduction in general and cardiovascular mortality and a reduction in infarctions in the first, second and third year, while sudden death was curbed only in the first year. No change in non-fatal infarctions was registered. It was not possible to establish whether these results were directly related to physical activity or also to other associated treatments. Therefore, there is still no definite evidence that physical activity and sports practice alone can determine an increase in survival and a change in coronary events in subjects suffering from ischemic cardiopathy, although they may certainly contribute alongside other treatments to an effective secondary prevention.

How Coronary Heart Disease Patients should Practice Sports

Some reports of sudden death or infarction occurring during sports practice and the rare incidents that have occurred during ergometric tests indicate that physical exercise can indeed be harmful to subjects suffering from ischemic heart disease. From this we can infer that sports practice cannot be recommended indiscriminately.

The sports practiced by coronary heart disease patients must have specific characteristics and must be carried out following specific rules.

Sports practice must first of all be tolerated with respect to the functional cardiac conditions, it must be enjoyed by patients, it must entail a sufficient but not excessive metabolic load (< 5-7 mets) and, furthermore, it should be measurable and prevalently aerobic.

Advice on the sport to practice must be preceded by a functional assessment test, after which the patient must be checked during and after the specific sports activity. Competitive sports or sports requiring static efforts and psychological excitement should be avoided. Also team sports in which it is difficult to assess energy expenditure are not recommended. Furthermore, exercise should be avoided after meals and in bad weather conditions (temperature, humidity, altitude). Sports that can be practised by and recommended to ischemic heart disease patients are: walking or jogging up to 6 km/h, cycling on flat surfaces up to 16 km/h, gymnastics, golf, tennis (doubles), horseback riding (lope and trot), cross-country skiing on flat surfaces up to 6 km/h, rowing up to 6 km/h, swimming up to 30 m/min.

In the light of the above considerations, it is falt that ischemic heart disease patients are also covered by the criteria described in 1980 in the Guideline for Graded Exercise Testing and Exercise Prescription (2 Ed. Lea & Febiger - Philadelphia) which states: "people of any age can engage in considerable levels of physical activity providing there are no contra-indications and the programme is carried out in a rational way."

References

1. Morris ChK, Froelicher V F (1993) Cardiovascular benefits of improved exercise capacity Sports Med, 16:225-236
2. Amsterdam EA, Laslett LJ, Dressendorfer RH, Mason DT (1981) Exercise training in coronary heart disease: is there a cardiac effect? Am Heart J 101:870-873
3. Vecchio C, La Rovere MT (1981) Influenza della riabilitazione sulla storia naturale del soggetto infartuato. Giorn Ital Cardiol 11:671-678
4. Hulls SS, Vamoli E, Adamson PB, Verrier RI, Foreman RD, Shwartz PJ (1994) Exercise training confirms anticipatory protection from sudden death during acute myocardial ischemia. Circulation 89:548-552
5. Berg A, Frey I, Baumstarl MW, Halle M, Keul J (1994) Physical activity and lipoprotein disorders. Sports Med 17:6-21
6. Giada F, Baldo-Enzi G, Baiocchi R, Zuliani G, Vitale E, Fellin R (1991) Specialized physical training program: effect on serum lipoprotein cholesterol, apoproteins A-1 and B and lipolitic enzyme activities. J Sports Med and Phys Fitness 31:196-203
7. Pitscheider W, Erlicher A, Zammarchi A, Crepax R, Romeo C, Oberhollenzer R, Mantone A, Braito E (1995) Rimodellamento del ventricolo sinistro a tre mesi da un primo infarto transmurale: influenza dell'attività fisica e della pervietà dell'arteria di necrosi sulle modificazioni dei volumi e della cinetica segmentaria. Giorn Ital Cardiol 25:421-431
8. American College of Sports Medicine. Position stand the recommended quantity and quality of exercise for developing and maintaining cardiorespiratory and muscular fitness in healthy adults (1990) J Cardiopulmonary Rehabilitation 10:235-245

9. Mc Henry PL, Ellstad MH, Fletcher GF, Pollock M (1990) Statement on exercise Circulation 81:396-398
10. O'Connor GT, Buring JE, Yusuf S, Goldhaber SZ, Omstead EM, Paffenbarger RS, Hennekens CH (1989) An overview of randomized trials of rehabilitation with exercise after myocardial infarction. Circulation 80:234-244

Electrocardiographic Repolarization Abnormalities in Athletes

M. Penco

Department of Cardiology, University of L'Aquila, L'Aquila, Italy

Abnormalities of ventricular repolarization (AVR) represent one of the alterations that most frequently require a detailed assessment by the sports physician. Transitory modifications of the T wave and ST segment can also be found in varying degrees in sedentary subjects in many physiological conditions such as, for example, hyperventilation, postural changes, etc.

As far as abnormalities of the T wave present in sportsmen are concerned, these are found with a frequency varying from 0.5% in the general sports population to 18% in a more selected group; they are very often associated with a negative clinical and instrumental examination, and only in a minority of cases (about 10%) with an "extreme" cardiac hypertrophy evident at echocardiogram. The cardiac diseases most frequently associated with these abnormalities are mitral valve prolapse, hypertrophic cardiomyopathy, cardiomyopathies, especially right ventricular cardiomyopathy characterized by negative T waves in the right precordial leads, cardiac hyperkinetic syndrome and, much more rarely, conditions of volume or pressure overload of both ventricles due to valvular disease, congenital heart diseases or hypertension. ECG identification of these conditions requires complete clinical and instrumental assessment, including patient case-history, the clinical symptoms, an objective examination, single (M-mode) and two-dimensional (2D) echocardiogram and a maximal stress test.

The ST segment and T wave abnormalities present at rest but more evident during stress, or which appear exclusively under stress, are perhaps an even greater problem than AVR in resting conditions. First of all these should be distinguished into a more frequent form, represented by the so-called "premature repolarization" (an ST segment elevation present in at least two consecutive precordial leads, associated or not with modifications of the T wave), that may be found in up to 50% of an unselected athlete population and clearly related to their level of fitness, as demonstrated by their regression on discontinuation of physical activity or after sympathetic stimulation [1, 2]. Less frequent are the so-called "pseudoischaemic alterations" of the repolarization phase (types II and III of Taggart's classification) which concern a dyshomogeneity of ventricular repolarization due to modifications of neuroadrenergic tone by the sympathetic nerves of the cardiac system and/or by the level of circulating catecholamines with the possible involvement of genetic predisposition [3, 4]. Such abnormalities may be studied by performing tests of sympathetic stimulation (with and without drugs), as well as electrocardiographic examination during isotonic stress tests on the cycloergometer or treadmill. Actually, the limited specificity of the first approach and the well known limits of the second, in a population such as athletes, that has a low prevalence of illness in general, and of myocardial ischaemia in particular, and in which additional factors, such as cardiac hypertrophy from training, may be responsible for false positive results, noticeably alters the utility of these tests.

Similar considerations may be made for abnormalities of the ST segment during or after stress, not often found (9-10%), even if similar prevalence has been found in a population of asymptomatic male sedentary subjects [5].

In all the above cases there is a need for a clinical diagnostic test to identify any possible myocardial ischaemia, or that would exclude it with more reliable sensitivity and specificity than that provided by electrocardiographic examinations. Perfusional 201 T1 or 99 Tc-MIBI myocardial scintigraphy does not appear to be a sufficiently reliable test as it can reveal abnormalities of coronary perfusion distribution not necessarily associated with the presence of myocardial ischaemia [6]. However, studies carried out on groups of sportsmen show frequent perfusional defects that are not indicative of myocardial ischaemia and which are referred to as dyshomogeneous captation because of the increase in myocardial mass and/or the metabolic peculiarity of myocardial fibre cells in fit hearts [7]. These observations underscore the current lack of knowledge on the normal perfusional scintigraphies in athletes and, therefore, on the limits which exist between physiological and pathological findings. The need to use the expertise of a nuclear medicine laboratory, the high costs of these examinations, the necessity for suitable technical-methodological standards, as well as the not easy adoption of correct interpretative criteria, underline how these investigations should be reserved for very particular cases and only after other means of investigation in the clinical-diagnostic iter have already supplied suitable documentation of myocardial ischaemia.

In contrast, stress-echocardiographic imaging has diagnostic sensitivity and specificity that permit its application in the sports population to assess asymptomatic abnormalities of repolarization present at rest or appearing under stress [8, 9].

The low prevalence of coronary disease in the population of asymptomatic young people could mean a lower sensitivity than that found in symptomatic subjects, even if in this regard there is no data relative to an appropriate number of persons. Extremely useful for clinical reasons is the integration of reversible wall motion abnormalities, an extremely specific marker of myocardial ischaemia, the results being supplied by ECG. The high specificity and therefore the reduced occurrence of false positives appears to be particularly advantageous, especially in sportsmen and women over 35-40 years of age; a population continuously increasing in number.

The possible detection of coronary artery disease in patients with acute coronary ischaemic syndromes that occur during sports activities and/or the autoptic findings of heart disease in subjects aged over 35 years who die suddenly, outline the potential of stress echocardiography for the screening of asymptomatic subjects in so-called "risk" age groups who are regularly engaged in physical activity [10-12]. In this population the detection of indicative markers of silent ischaemia would be extremely useful to identify subjects with unidentified coronary artery disease. At present, on the basis of clinical application of Bayes' theorem, this population has a low occurrence of heart disease. The predictive accuracy of stress echocardiography, although not sufficiently investigated, seems too low to indicate wide use of this method in the screening of asymptomatic subjects, the some finding as for stress electrocardiography.

Despite the current diffusion of the method, many authors still believe that stress echocardiography is a procedure "for experts", to be limited to a few laboratories able to obtain high quality images and to get the best results from this technique. Even if so up to a few years ago, the method appears to have been remarkably changed by the widespread marketing of computerizing imaging systems. In fact, in recent years the use of stress echocardiography has become widely established and is gaining increasing approval in its specific application of sports cardiology.

More recently, the limitations associated with the difficulties in performing a correct echocardiographic examination during physical exercise and/or the lack of attaining a suitable working load have led to the introduction of the so-called "alternative stresses" into clinical practice. These stresses, especially used in the diagnosis of myocardial ischaemia, have the main objective of obviating the limitations of physical exercise and of inducing ischaemia through increasing oxygen myocardial requests (atrial pacing for a prevalent increase in heart rate, catecholamine, especially dobutamine, for a prevalent inotropic stimulation and, in a lesser way, of the heart rate). Ischaemia can also be induced by a modification in the intracoronary distribution of myocardial flow with induction of ischaemia through the mechanism of "vertical" or "horizontal" steal (dipyridamole, adenosyne, etc.).

However, echocardiography during pharmacological stress has not found extensive application in the field of sports cardiology and, in our opinion, in the population of subjects who practice sports activities the use of physical stress appears more justified.

In conclusion, the use of stress echocardiography should not be confined only to the study of ischaemic heart disease. Such an approach would be too restrictive to the capabilities of a method so suitable for the diagnostic definition of ventricular repolarization abnormalities sometimes accompanied by the painful precordial symptoms but more often quite asymptomatic.

References

1. Zehender M, Meinertz T, Keul J, Just H (1990) ECG variants and cardiac arrythmias in athletes: clinical relevance and prognostic importance. Am Heart J 119:1378
2. Oakley DG, Oakley CM (1982) Significance of abnormal electrocardiograms in highly trained athletes. Am J Cardiol 50:985

3. Serra Grima JS, Carrio I, Estorch M, Gaya G, Pons G, Varas C, Bayes De Luna A (1986) ECG alterations in the athlete type ìpseudoischemiaî. Int J Sports Card 3:9
4. Taggart P, Carruthers M, Joseph S, Kelly HB, Marcomichelakis J, Noble D, O'Neill G, Somerville W (1979) Electrocardiographic changes resembling myocardial ischemia in asymptomatic men with normal coronary arteriograms. Br Heart J 41:214
5. Spirito P, Maron BJ, Bonow RO, Epstein SE (1983) Prevalence and significance of a abnormal ST segment response to exercise in a young athletic population. Am J Cardiol 51:1663
6. Schwartz RS, Jackson WG, Celio PV, Richardson LA, Hickman JR jr (1993) Accuracy of exercise 201 Tl myocardial scintigraphy in asymptomatic young men. Circulation 87:165
7. Osbakken M, Locko R (1984) Scintigraphic determination of ventricular function and coronary perfusion in long-distance runners. Am Heart J 108:296
8. Dagianti A, Penco M, Agati L, Sciomer S, Dagianti A jr, Rosanio S, Fedele F (1995) Stress echocardiography: comparison of exercise, dipyridamole and dobutamine in detecting and predicting the extent of coronary artery disease. J Am Coll Cardiol 26:18
9. Douglas PS, OíToole ML, Woolard J (1990) Regional wall motion abnormalities after prolonged exercise in the normal left ventricle. Circulation 82:2108
10. Ciampricotti R, El Gamal M, Relik T, Taverne R, Panis J, de Swart J, vanGelder B, vanWely L (1990) Clinical characteristics and coronary angiographic findings of patients with unstable angina, acute myocardial infarction and survivors of sudden ischemic death occurring during and after sport. Am Heart J 120:1267
11. Waller BF, Roberts WC (1980) Sudden death while running in conditioned runners aged 40 years or over. Am J Cardiol 45:1292
12. Liberthson RR (1996) Sudden death from cardiac causes in children and young adults. New Engl J Med 334 (16):1039

Arterial Hypertension and Physical Activity

R. H. Fagard

Hypertension and Cardiovascular Rehabilitation Unit, Dpt. of Molecular and Cardiovascular Research, Faculty of Medicine, Univ. of Leuven, K.U.L., Leuven, Belgium

Scientific evidence suggests that there is a mutual relationship between blood pressure and physical activity. On one hand, a high blood pressure may adversely affect exercise performance, on the other dynamic exercise training seems to contribute to the control of blood pressure. These relationships between pressure and activity will be explored in this review.

Blood Pressure and Maximal Exercise Capacity

There is quite some evidence that a high blood pressure is associated with a lower peak oxygen uptake [1]. In patients with mild essential hypertension peak oxygen uptake for graded bicycle exercise was 20% lower [2] and the tolerance for progressive treadmill exercise 17% lower [3] than in age- and sex-matched healthy normotensive controls. Amery et al [4] found that the maximal oxygen uptake of hypertensive patients was not significantly impaired when compared to normotensives, but a decline occurred with increasing severity of hypertension within the hypertensive group. Similarly, in 50 young and middle-aged untreated men with essential hypertension and limited organ damage (WHO stages I or II), peak oxygen uptake on graded uninterrupted bicycle exercise was inversely related to mean intra-arterial pressure at rest (Fig 1), but also to age [5]. In multiple regression analysis factors such as blood pressure, age and weight contributed independently to the variation in maximal oxygen uptake. In addition, men with hypertension had a greater decrease of estimated peak oxygen uptake per kilogram body weight with age than normal men [6]. Several data suggest that not blood pressure per se, but long-term consequences of hypertension, which are not necessarily clinically apparent, could be responsible for the reduction of aerobic power. When adolescents were studied peak oxygen uptake was similar in subjects with sustained essential hypertension, youngsters with labile hypertension and age-matched normotensive controls [7]. Also Wilson et al [8] observed that boys with persistently elevated blood pressures had normal fitness, but aerobic power was decreased in girls with elevated pressures. When patients with obesity and echocardiographic abnormalities were excluded in a study on adults, oxygen consumption at peak exercise was similar in normotensives, mildly hypertensives and more severe hypertensives [9]. In hypertensive patients without heart failure, echocardiographic left

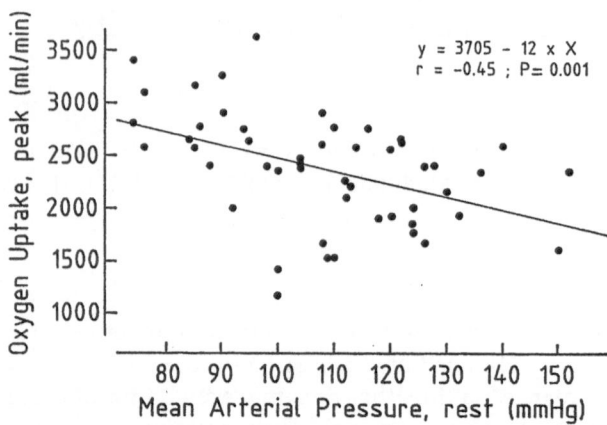

Fig. 1. Relation between peak oxygen uptake (ml/min) and mean intra-arterial brachial artery pressure at supine rest (mmHg) in male patients referred for hypertension. The relation remains significant after adjustment for age and weight (From Fagard, RH. Maximal aerobic power in essential hypertension. Journal of Hypertension 1988, 6:859-856 (Fig. 1))

ventricular mass or fractional fiber shortening at rest were not related to the time that graded exercise could be sustained [3]. However, hemodynamic measurements during exercise revealed a shift of the cardiac function curve to the right in the patients with the highest blood pressure, as compared to age-matched patients with less severe hypertension, suggesting that impairment of cardiac function without clinical heart failure could be involved [5]. Exercise capacity was clearly impaired after the development of overt heart failure [3]. Finally, maximal exercise testing evoked no impairment in younger patients with increased blood pressure, but showed progressively greater impairment in older patients with higher levels of hypertension, left ventricular hypertrophy, retinopathy and coronary artery disease [10].

Influence of Physical Training on Blood Pressure

Many studies have been performed on the effect of dynamic physical training on blood pressure. The present overview will be restricted to controlled studies on the effect of dynamic physical training on blood pressure, which involved adolescent or adult normotensive and or hypertensive subjects in whom cardiovascular diseases were reasonably well excluded. Details of the 36 reports and the main findings of the overall analysis of the 48 study groups have been published before [11, 12]. Most of the participants were men and the average age of the groups ranged from 16 to 72 years. Duration of training ranged from 4 to 68 weeks (median = 16 weeks), with a frequency of mostly 3 weekly sessions of 15 to 90 minutes each; training intensity was between 50 and 85% of maximal exercise testing. Table 1 summarizes the training-induced changes, weighted for the number of participants in each group and adjusted for the control data. The significant increase in physical work capacity and decrease in heart rate demonstrate the overall efficacy of the training programs. Blood pressure was significantly lowered by an average of 5.3/4.8 mmHg for systolic and diastolic pressure respectively. The response of blood pressure was not related to the change in body weight (P > 0.50), which averaged -0.84 kg.

Table 1. Training-induced changes (weighted means, adjusted for control data) and 95% confidence limits of systolic and diastolic blood pressure at rest, heart rate at rest, body weight and physical work capacity (PWC), of all study groups combined; the number refers to the number of study groups for which the variable was reported.

	Net weighted mean	95% confidence limits	Number of groups
Blood pressure (mmHg)			
systolic	- 5.3	- 7.2; - 3.4	48
diastolic	- 4.8	- 6.2; - 3.4	47
Heart rate (min^{-1})	- 6.1	- 7.3; - 4.8	36
Weight (kg)	-0.84	-1.16; -0.53	35
PWC (%)	+15.1	+13.4; +16.9	43

(From Fagard RH. The role of exercise in blood pressure control. Journal of Hypertension 1995, 13:1223-1227 (Tab. 1 and Fig. 1))

Results According to Baseline Blood Pressure

The response of blood pressure differed according to the pretraining blood pressure level. When the 48 study groups were classified into 3 categories by the average pretraining blood pressure according to the 1978 criteria of the World Health Organisation, dynamic training was associated with a mean net change (95% C.L.) of -3 (-5;-1) /-3 (-4;-2) mmHg in the 27 groups with a normal average pressure, -6 (-9;-3) /-7 (-11;-3) mmHg in borderline hypertensive patients (n = 7) and -10 (-14;-6) /-8 (-11;-4) mmHg in the hypertensive patients (n = 14). The suggestion that the response of blood pressure is more pronounced in the hypertensive patients is corroborated by the results of studies in which normotensive and hypertensive patients followed the same training program. In each of these studies the blood pressure change was greater in the hypertensive patients than in the normotensives; the weighted averages (95% C.L.) were - 13 (-15;-11) /-8 (-10;-6) mmHg in the hypertensives and -3 (-7;+0.5) /-2 (-5;+1) mmHg in the normotensives.

Results According to Study Design

The criteria for inclusion of studies in the present meta-analysis is open to criticism. First, allocation to the active or control group, or the order of the training and non-training periods was not always determined at random. Second, the subjects in the control group or in the control period were seldom seen as regularly as those in the training program or they were not followed up during

134   R. H. Fagard

control. In addition, it should be realized that it is difficult to blind the participants to the treatment in training studies; some authors included low level exercise as placebo-treatment. Figure 2 represents an attempt to analyse the results in 3 categories according to the study design. Several studies did not include a randomization procedure and in some randomly allocated studies the control subjects were seen only at the beginning and at the end of the control period. In others, allocation of the control group or the order of the periods was determined at random and the subjects in the control group or period were followed or contacted regularly. It can been seen in Figure 2 that studies which followed the more rigorous scientific criteria showed the smallest decrease in blood pressure, which was not significant in normotensives but still significant in the hypertensive patients, that is -7/-5 mmHg for systolic and diastolic pressure respectively.

Results on Ambulatory Blood Pressure

Another major criticism of the reviewed studies is that few mention that the investigator who measured the blood pressure was unaware of the treatment group or period and that special methodologies such as a random-zero sphygmomanometry, non-portable automated devices or intra-arterial measurements were not often used for the blood pressure measurement. This problem can be overcome to some extent by the use of ambulatory monitoring devices. Though the number of studies is still limited [12], the results indicate that day-

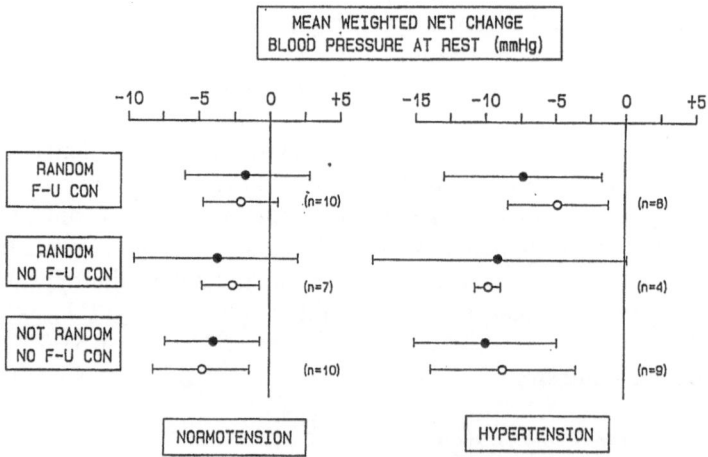

Fig. 2. The training-induced changes of blood pressure and 95% confidence limits (mmHg), in normotensives and hypertensives, weighted for the number of participants and adjusted for control data, according to the study design. Random: studies which included a randomization procedure; F-U: studies which included some follow-up of the subjects in the control group or period (From Fagard RH. The role of exercise in blood pressure control. Journal of Hypertension 1995, 13:1223-1227 (Tab. 1 and Fig. 1))

time systolic pressure does not decrease when its baseline level is below 140 mm Hg; the few reports with baseline blood pressure above this level suggest that physical training may induce a hypotensive response in these subjects. Similarly, decreases of daytime diastolic blood pressure seem to be restricted to groups with the higher baseline diastolic pressure. By contrast, nighttime pressure did not change significantly, except for diastolic pressure in one study in hypertensive patients. The lack of an effect during sleep, when sympathetic activity is low, is compatible with the suggestion that sympathetic withdrawal contributes to the antihypertensive effect of training.

Further Limitations of the Training Studies

Other shortcomings include the fact that advice to keep diet and/or lifestyle constant throughout the study periods was only given in half of the studies; diet was controlled by interviews in about a quarter of the reports and 24-h urinary sodium excretion was assessed in a similar number. The percentage of included subjects who could not be analysed at the end of the study was less than 70% in one fifth of the study groups. As for the statistical analysis, most authors reported the significance of the response in the trained group and in the controls separately; the significance of the difference between the changes in the 2 groups was given in less than half of the studies. Furthermore, adjustment for confounding variables such as changes in weight was not often performed.

Practical Recommendations

Because of the possible beneficial effects of exercise on blood pressure, other cardiovascular risk factors, morbidity and mortality adequate progressive dynamic physical training is advocated for the management of hypertensive patients, together with nonpharmacologic measures in the mild hypertensive or as an adjunct to pharmacologic treatment in more severe hypertensive patients. Because hypertension is a risk factor for cardiovascular morbidity and mortality, an exercise test may be recommended in addition to the regular work-up, in previously sedentary patients, particularly when other risk factors such as smoking, obesity or hyperlipidemia are present or when the patient complains of dyspnea or chest pain [13].

When hypertension is detected in an athlete [14] a screening investigation is warranted including history, physical examination, electrocardiography, echocardiography, exercise testing, eye-ground examination, urine analysis, blood hemoglobin, blood glucose, renal function, serum electrolytes and cholesterol. The decision to perform further examinations to exclude secondary forms of hypertension are based on the results of the screening tests, the severity of hypertension and the presence of target organ damage. Further management has to be guided according to conventional guidelines, such as the 1993 recommendations of WHO/ISH [15]. The athlete should be treated by selected pharmacologic means when there is no doubt that this is beneficial; in areas of doubt, a waiting attitude is justified because 1) hypertension has not been associated with sudden death in the young athlete, and 2) there is no evidence that sports affects the prognosis unfavorably. High level sports activity can be allowed when blood pressure is controlled and when it is not precluded or rendered unwise by severe target organ damage or an underlying illness. Prescription of antihypertensive drugs should take into account the possible negative effects of diuretics, at least during short term-treatment, and particularly of beta-blockers on exercise performance [1].

Acknowledgements. The authors gratefully acknowledge the secretarial assistance of N. Ausseloos.

References

1. Fagard R, Amery A (1995) Physical exercise in hypertension. In: Hypertension: Pathophysiology, Diagnosis and Management, 2nd ed. Edited by Laragh JH, Brenner BM. Raven Press, Ltd., New York, pp 2669-2681
2. Missault L, Duprez D, de Buyzere M, de Backer G, Clement D (1992) Decreased exercise capacity in mild essential hypertension: non-invasive indicators of limiting factors. J Hum Hypertens 6:151-155
3. Ajayi AAL, Akinwusi PO (1993) Spectrum of hypertensive heart disease in Nigerians: cross sectional study of echocardiographic indices and their correlation with treadmill exercise capacity. J Hypertens 11:99-102
4. Amery A, Julius S, Whitlock LS, Conway J (1967) Influence of hypertension on the hemodynamic response to exercise. Circulation 36:231-237
5. Fagard R, Staessen J, Amery A (1988) Maximal aerobic power in essential hypertension. J Hypertens 6:859-865
6. Bruce RA, Fisher LD, Cooper MN, Gey GO (1974) Separation of effects of cardiovascular disease and age on ventricular function with maximal exercise. Am J Cardiol 34:757-763
7. Nudel DB, Gootman N, Brunson SC, Stenzler A, Shenker IR, Gauthier BG (1980) Exercise performance of hypertensive adolescents. Pediatrics 65:1073-1078
8. Wilson SL, Gaffney FA, Laird WP, Fixler DE (1985) Body size, composition, and fitness in adolescents with elevated blood pressure. Hypertension 7:417-422
9. Agostoni P, Doria E, Berti M, Alimento M, Tamborini G, Fiorentini C (1992) Exercise performance in patients with uncomplicated essential hypertension. Chest 101:1591-1596
10. Wong HE, Kasser IS, Bruce RA (1969) Impaired maximal exercise performance with hypertensive cardiovascular disease. Circulation 39:633-638
11. Fagard RH, Tipton CM. Physical activity, fitness and hypertension. In: Physical activity, fitness and health. International Proceedings and Consensus Statement. Edited by Bouchard C, Shephard RJ, Stephens T (1994) Human Kinetics Publishers Inc., Champaign IL pp 633-655
12. Fagard RH (1993) The role of exercise in blood pressure control: supportive evidence. J Hypertens 13:1223-1227
13. Fagard RH (1995) Prescription and results of physical activity. J Cardiovasc Pharmacol 25 (Suppl 1):S20-S27

14. Kaplan NM, Devereux R, Miller HS (1994) Systemic hypertension. In: Recommendations for determining eligibility for competition in athletes with cardiovascular abnormalities. Med Sci Sports Ex 26 (Suppl 10):S268-S270
15. Guidelines for the management of mild hypertension: memorandum from a WHO /ISH meeting (1993) J Hypertension 11:905-918

Arterial and Venous Diseases in Athletes

L. Pedrini, F. Magnoni

Dept. of Vascular Surgery, Maggiore C.A. Pizzardi Hospital, Bologna, Italy,

Vascular diseases in fit young athletes are rare. The lifestyle and metabolic modifications induced by physical activity reduce the risk of atherosclerotic lesions; likewise, muscular activity improves venous outflow.

The vascular lesions observed after bone or joint traumas are seldom caused by sports and resemble those caused by other factors. Similarly, traumatic injuries of blood vessels are occasionally observed in sports, but rarely can they be considered a particular risk of a specific sport.

Most vascular lesions in athletes are caused by recurrent microvascular injuries. Anatomical abnormalities, muscular hypertrophy or static modifications of the shoulder or the spine concur to produce these lesions.

Sport may disclose the symptoms of a vascular disease at a younger age, but rarely is it the main etiology of a vascular lesion.

To simplify the description, vascular lesions have been classified in relation to the anatomical location and etiologic mechanism.

Upper Limbs

The most common pathology observed in athletes and in young people is the Thoracic Outlet Syndrome (TOS). All shoulder girdle compression syndromes have in common the compression of the brachial plexus and subclavian artery and vein, usually between the clavicle and the first rib (costoclavicular compression) [1]. Other common causes of vascular compression are:
- scalenus anticus hypertrophy or anomaly
- cervical rib and/or fibrous band
- outcome of clavicle or rib injury
- pectoralis minor muscle
- humeral head

Nerve symptoms are the most frequent, followed by venous signs, which range from edema, stiffness of the fingers and venous engorgement in certain elevated positions to acute thrombosis of the subclavian or axillary vein (effort vein thrombosis or Paget von Schroetter syndrome). Intermittent symptoms often precede the onset of acute thrombosis and can be observed both at night and after training or a match [2].

Arterial symptoms range from coolness, cold sensitivity and pallor of the hand on elevation to a fully developed Raynaud's phenomenon. Acute ischemia can be observed after the occlusion of the subclavian artery or after arterial embolism due to a post-stenotic aneurysm of the subclavian artery. A cervical rib is the most frequent cause of this lesion (Fig. 1). In many cases a thrombolytic therapy must be performed in the acute phase, before the treatment of the compression or vascular reconstruction.

TOS has been observed in many sports involving the upper limbs (baseball, kayak, weight lifting, basket-ball, volley-ball) [3, 4].

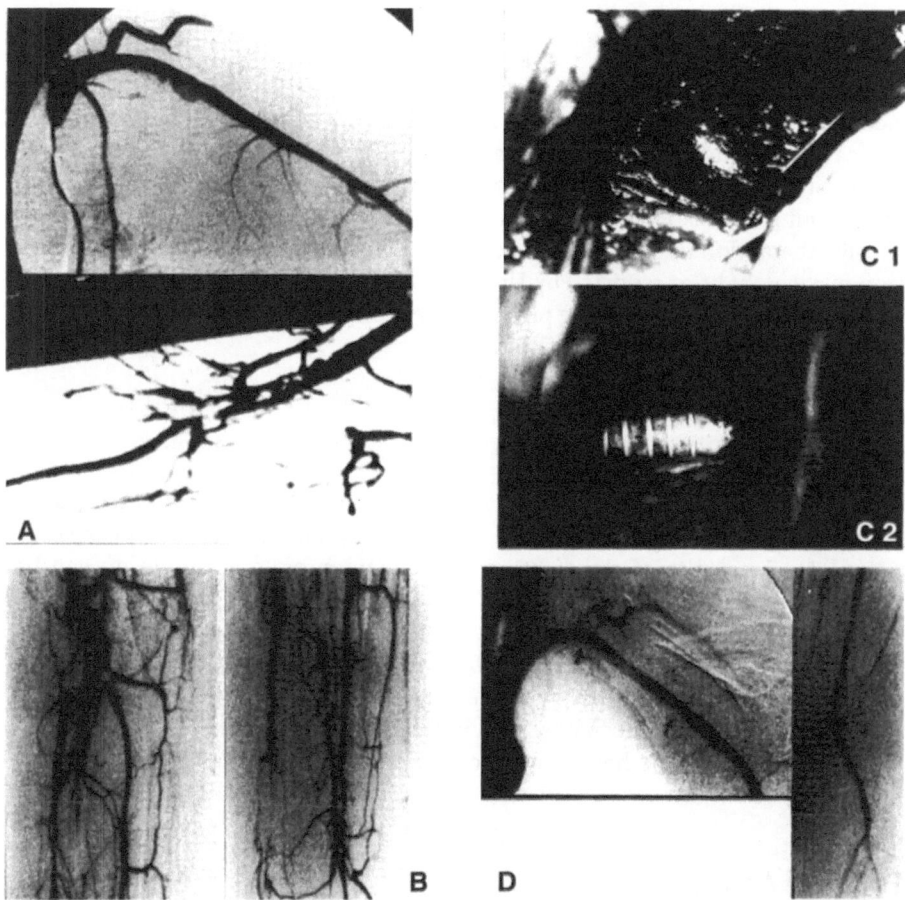

Fig. 1. Critical hand ischemia in a volley-ball player, with symptoms raised more than 15 days before admission. **a)** pre-treatment angiography: subclavian artery aneurysm with embolic occlusion of the brachial, radial and ulnar arteries. **b)** angiograpy performed after 24 hours of intra-arterial thrombolysis with urokinase (40,000 I.U./hour).
c) intraoperative view: subclavian artery aneurysm (**c1**) repaired by a ringed PTFE graft after the excision of the cervical rib (**c2**) **d)** post-treatment angiography: complete restoration of arterial patency after aneurysm resection and thrombectomy of brachial, ulnar and radial arteries

Hand Ischemia

Hand ischemia can be linked to arterial embolism but is more frequently secondary to repeated microtraumas with digital or palmar artery occlusion. It is a complication of many sports such as volley-ball, hand-ball, pelota, baseball and frisbee. [4, 5].

Symptoms range from Raynaud's phenomenon to acute ischemia or gangrene of one or more fingers and are exacerbated by frequent abnormalities of the superficial or deep palmar arch [6].

Aortic Dissection

Acute aortic dissection has been observed in many athletes and has often been the cause of sudden death during a match. It is more frequent in basket-ball players (tall men with a constitution similar to patients with Marfan's syndrome), but it has also been described during skiing practice [7]. Dissection may involve the abdominal aorta or a peripheral artery as in a case of iliac dissection in a weight lifter reported by Urbano et al [8].

Hypertensive spikes during physical stress can be responsible for the dissection in patients with medial degeneration.

Iliac Artery

Stenotic intimal thickening of the external iliac artery has been described in young competition cyclists [9] and in amateurs, whose lesions appear some years later. Intermittent claudication is the main symptom; the lesion can be confirmed by duplex scanning.

One of the patho-physiological theories proposed suggests the involvement of many factors such as an increased flow, the sitting position of the cyclist and the links of the end of this artery to the pelvis caused by its lateral branches.

A similar lesion has been observed in long distance runners. [10]

Iliac artery stenosis has been described even in a 28 year old male rugby player [11] but in this case a post-traumatic etiology was implicated.

Popliteal Artery

The popliteal artery entrapment syndrome is a vascular complication observed more frequently in athletes than in people who do not practise sport.

An abnormal insertion of the medial head of the gastrocnemius muscle is the main cause, but compression due to the tendon of gracilis, the popliteal or plantaris muscle, Baker's cysts or muscular hypertrophy have been reported. In an early stage intermittent claudication is the main symptom, but unfortunately many patients have been observed after a thrombotic or embolic complication. Venous or nervous compression may be associated and in these cases pain, paresthesias, sensation of tension or edema have been reported.

Also in these cases sport is responsible for muscular hypertrophy which is why athletes complain of symptoms at a younger age.

Varicose Veins

Muscular activity increases blood flow, which is responsible for the engorgement of the superficial veins in athletes. These veins cannot be considered varicose veins because they are linear and their valves have normal function.

Varicose veins of the lower limbs are observed in about 5% of practising athletes, notably weight-lifters and wrestlers, but also in karate, judo, canoeing, soccer and high jump [12], possibly in people with an anatomical predisposition to varicose veins.

Popliteal Vein

A venous compression of the popliteal vein due to a narrow solear ring has been described by Servelle. The symptoms of this syndrome are leg heaviness, edema, varicosis of the intersaphenic veins or deep venous thrombosis.

Muscular hypertrophy causes a further narrowing of this space and venous compression. We observed a solear syndrome in a high jumper, who complained of acute edema of the leg after a competition, phlebography disclosed a compression of the tibio-peroneal trunk induced by the dorsal flexion of the foot.

Conclusions

In conclusion, vascular complications in athletes can involve arteries and veins in any site, but they are rare. Adson [13] in 1947 reported that he had "never been called on to operate on athletes, wrestlers, boxers or football players with marked muscular hypertrophy or with heavy descending shoulders" probably because a "person who has these congenital anomalies learned early in life that it was painful to pursue vigorous activity and therefore avoided athletics". Nevertheless, the number of persons who practice sports is so great that some will crop up in the experience of vascular surgeons.

Trainers and medical doctors should be aware of these possible hazards in order to avoid the serious complications; vascular laboratory and imaging will be useful to confirm the diagnosis and to choose the correct treatment.

References

1. Roos DB, Owens C (1966) Thoracic outlet syndrome. Arch Surg 93:71-4
2. D'Addato M, Curti T, Paragona O (1983) La sindrome da ostacolato scarico venoso nello sportivo. Med sport 36(6):481-8
3. Rohrer MJ, Cardullo PA, Pappas AM, Phillips DA, Wheeler HB (1990) Axillary artery compression and thrombosis in throwing athletes. J Vasc Surg 11:761-9
4. McCarthy WJ, Yao JST, Schafer MF, Nuber G, Flinn WR, Blackburn D, Suker JR (1989) Upper extremity arterial injury in athletes. J Vasc Surg 9:317-327
5. Curti T, Pedrini L, Cifiello Bl, Saccà A (1984) Vasculopatie della mano e trauma da sport. Min Angiol 9(3):365-6
6. Pedrini L, Pilla G, Saccà A (1983) Arcate vascolari palmari: variazioni anatomiche. Riv Chir Mano XX(1): 115-7
7. Calamai G, Alajmo F, Montesi G, Braconi L, Vaccari G, Gori A (1993) Dissezione aortica acuta in corso di pratica dello sci in due pazienti. Possibili implicazioni chirurgiche. Arch Chir Torac Cardiovasc 15:519-22
8. Urbano O, Luca A, Quartuccio S, La Spada M, Carella I, Romeo P, Spinelli F, Longo FN (1992) Su un caso di dissecazione dell'iliaca Dx in giovane pesista. Min Angiol 17(Suppl 1 al N° 2):137
9. Rousselet MC, Saint-Andre JP, L'Hoste P, Enon B, Megret A, Chevalier JM (1990) Stenotic intimal thickening of the external iliac artery in competition cyclists. Hum Pathol 21:524-9
10. Gallegos CRR, Studley JGN, Hamer DB (1989) External iliac artery occlusion: another complication of long distance running. Eur J Vasc Surg 4: 195-6
11. Bray AE, Lewis WA (1992) Intermittent claudication in a professional rugby player. J Vasc Surg 15:664-8
12. Venerando A, Pelliccia A (1981) Physiopathologie de la circulation veineuse superficielle des athlèts. Phlébologie 34(2):289-298
13. Adson M (1947) Surgical treatment for symptoms produced by cervical ribs and the scalenus anticus muscle. Surg Gynec Obst 85:687-700

Noncardiac Diseases Mimicking and/or Affecting the Cardiovascular System

G. Caldarone, R. Lista

Department of Medicine, Institute of Sport Sciences, Rome, Italy

It is well known that diseases of the cardiovascular system constitute the most frequent cause of morbidity and mortality in industrialized countries as well as the most frequent cause of hospitalization and invalidity. In the case of a young athlete who presents cardiovascular symptomatology, the first suspicion is a cardiac cause; this has notable psychological implication in the subject and it makes a precise and timely clinical solution important. In fact, we often find young subjects in good general health and physically very active in whom a contingent diagnosis of cardiopathy would gravely limit or interrupt sporting activity. Therefore, a careful and correct general clinical evaluation, a specific clinical and instrumental heart evaluation and a good knowledge of the intensity and the degree of physical effort that the athlete is undergoing when the symptom develop, is of utmost importance. The principal and most frequent noncardiac clinical situation, but in which the cardiovascular system seems involved, are described below.

Symptoms that Could Affect Cardiac Pathologies in Athletes

Main confounding symptoms are:
- chest pain
- asthenia and easy tiring
- dyspnea
- palpitations
- lipothymia and syncope

Chest pain is one of the typical symptomatologic manifestations of various cardiopathies. However, chest pain represents an alarming event even when it originates from alterations of other organs and systems, in particular the respiratory system, the osteoarticular system, muscular and radicular structures of the thorax and of the neck and the gastrointestinal system.

Cardiovascular causes	Non cardiovascular causes
Angina in its various forms	Muscoloskeletal pain
Myocardial infarction	
Mitral valve prolapse	Cervical radiculopathy
Aortic dissection	Joint pain (painful shoulder: bursitis
	Rotator cuff injury, biceps tendinopathy)
	Costochondral (Tietze d.) and Xiphoid pain
	Pleural pain
	Pleuritis
	Pneumothorax
	Mediastinic emphysema
	Gastroenteric disease
	Gastroesophageal reflux disease
	Cholecystitis with or without calculuses
	Peptic ulcerous disease
	Pancreatitis
	Pulmonary disease
	Pulmonary hypertension
	Pneumonia
	Pulmonary embolism

Esophageal pathology represents the most common cause of non-cardiac thoracic pain, it is caused by distinctive defects of position of the esophagogastric junction such as the sliding hiatal hernia. In this pathologic condition, characterized by the reflux of small amounts of gastric juice into the esophageal mucous membrane, the clinical manifestations are prevalently heartburn, dysphagia and retrosternal pain. The pain from abnormal stimulation of the sensory nerve endings of the damaged esophageal mucous membrane causes a painful thoracic symptomatology that could make difficult a differential diagnosis with pain of cardiac origin.

Asthenia and Easy Fatigability

Cardiovascular causes	Non cardiovascular causes
Ischemic cardiopathy	Hypokinetic disease
Cardiomyopathy	Depression (it could be the first symptom)
Myocarditis	Cushing disease
Valvular alterations	Lupus (it could be the first symptom)
Pulmonary hypertension	Fever
Congenital heart diseases	Hyperthyroidism
Pericardial diseases	Anemia
Rhythm alterations (A-V block, etc.)	Oxide carbon intoxication
Congenital cardiopathy with shunt	

The athlete frequently reports an easier fatigability that he generally describes as a difficulty in finishing the training session. Such problems are rather frequent and generally appear in all the situations of malaise that can affect young people and sportsmen in particular. Viral infections are among the most common causes: they often run, particularly in the initial stage with short symptomatology, but they are always accompanied by "asthenia", this symptom becomes limiting especially when the person is subjected to intense physical activity.

Dyspnea

Dyspnea could be defined a general way as an abnormal and disagreeable awareness of breathing. It is a strictly subjective feeling. Effort dyspnea is the classical form of dyspnea of cardiac origin and is often the first manifestation of cardiac inadequacy or of inadequate cardiac output. Sometimes in sports-medicine athletes have reported difficulty in performing ample respiratory movements as if the subject feels an impediment to finish the breath. This symptom often coincides with a state of neurotic anxiety, or more generally could be part of an "overtraining" syndrome sometimes considered in high level athletes.

Lipothymias and Syncope

Cardiovascular causes	Non cardiovascular causes
Aortic stenosis	Hypoglycemia
Hypertrophic cardiomiopathy	Hyperventilation
Pulmonary embolism	Hysteria
Cardiac tumors	Acute dyspepsia
Cardiac tamponade	Prodromial phase of viral syndromes
	Heat stroke
Myocardial infarction	
Heart's rupture	
Tachycardia	
Bradycardia	
Sinus arrest or sinoatrial block	
Carotid sinus syndrome	
Complete (A-V block, etc.)	
Vascular peripheral Syncope	
Orthostatic hypotension, vaso-vagal	
Syncope	

Syncope is a sudden and momentary loss of conscience; while lipothymia (that could forestall a real fainting episode) never involves a real loss of conscience but consists of a sudden feeling of faint, light headedness and dizziness. It is not infrequent that sports persons also those trained to intense physical efforts should experience episodes of momentary loss of conscience like lipothymia or syncope. Such phenomena could be brought on by situations of not perfect well being, such as digestive disorders or in the prodromal symptoms of a viral illness. In this case the physical effort represent the provocative cause of the lipothymia and/or syncope.

Palpitations

Cardiovascular causes	Non cardiovascular causes
Arrhythmias	Hyperthyroidism
Miocarditis	Anxietly
	Hyperpyrexia
	Major physical efforts
	Accession of amphetaminic substances

Palpitations do not necessarily mean that the subject has a cardiac arrhythmia; infact they are a more frequent symptom in non cardiopathy subjects with states of distinctive nervous system excitability (for example in hyperthyroidism and in anxiety states) than in many patients with organic, even severe, cardiopathy. Therefore, they may have a quite benign meaning or represent alarm symptoms predictive of sudden death. Many non cardiac causes such as hyperpyrexia, consumption of amphetaminic substances, anemia, hyperventilation, hypoglycemia, anxiety crises and major a physical efforts could determine reported symptoms like alterations of the cardiac rhythm. Therefore it is essential to give ample space to a complete and accurate anamnesis.

Internal Diseases that Could Interest Cardiovascular System in Athlete

Athletes could become ill with chiefly non cardiac pathologies but which in their course could involve the cardiovascular system to varying degrees. This cardiac involvment could for some disease become the dominant element of the clinical picture.

Viral syndromes
Arterial hypertension
Hyperthyroidism and Hypothyroidism
Diabetes
Overweight and obesity
Drugs - doping substances
Marfan's disease
Electrolyte imbalances

Viral Syndromes:
Influenza syndrome, recurrent viral infections of the primary airway of the respiratory tract (rhinovirus) and acute infections of the gastrointestinal tract (enterovirus) are frequent in young athletes. A greater risk probably exists in

these subjects compared to sedentary subjects of the same age because of numerous aggravating factors in the sportsman (cold exposure, life in community, rapid changes of environmental temperature etc.) and because of increased decadence of the body's immune system in occasion of repeated and prolonged physical effort. In the course of these viral syndromes cardiocirculatory symptoms (palpitations, deep asthenia, lipothymias etc.) and ECG alterations of rhythm (myocardial involvment in the same viral disease) could appear. Viral incoming episodes can sometimes interest the young athlete and cause a sort of immunodeficiency syndrome frequently interpreted as "overtraining" syndrome.

Hypertension:
It is possible that high level athletes present high blood pressure values but trained to notable entity work loads. In these cases the evaluation of the subject has two principal objectives: to identify secondary forms of hypertension and to determine the presence of hypertensive damage to other organs or systems. For a detailed explanatión of the of the criteria to be followed in athletes, see chapter "Arterial Hypertension".

Thyroid Function Disorders:
The cardiac effects of alterations in thyroid function could arise from an excessive or insufficient direct action of the thyroid hormones on the heart, or from the extracardiac action of the same thyroid hormones and their effects, particularly on lipid metabolism. Palpitations and dyspnea are frequent symptoms in hyperthyroidism. In hipothyroidism there are apposite cardiovascular haemodynamic modifications accompanied by bradycardia and reduction of the cardiac course.

Diabetes:
The cardiovascular system constitutes the first target in both insulin-dependent and non insulin-dependent diabetes. In this pathologic condition there can be alterations of the small vessels (diabetic microangiopathy with involvement of capillaries, arterioles and venules); alterations of the large vessels (with the histologic appearance of atherosclerosis) and maybe also alterations to "diabetic type" cardiomyopathy.

Overweight and Obesity:
Besides being associated with increased incidence of arterial hypertension (up to 50% of obese patients have elevated blood pressure values) and alterations of lipid and glucose metabolism, with increased risk of coronary disease, overweight and obesity also determine several hemodynamic modifications. The increase of the fat mass is linked to a proportionate increase in blood volume and cardiac output. These factors, if persistent, induce a chronic volume overload of the left ventricle.

Cardiovascular Symptom Induced by Drugs and Doping Substances

Finally one must remember the cardiovascular alterations that can be induced both by drugs that are commonly thought to have express action on the cardiovascular system, and by substances some sportsmen use by in order to improve performance (doping). These represent a not insignificant event in clinical practice as: the "cardiovascular" effects of certain drugs are generally less known and so the of practice of doping is often not declared. The adverse reactions to the heart are essentially alterations of contractility and/or cardiac rhythm; some could cause angina crises particularly in patients with reduced coronary reserve. Among these drugs are:

- psychodrugs eg. tricyclic antidepressants (induce a sensitization to catecholamines with consequent orthostatic hypotension and disturbances of conduction and of rhythm)
- caffeine (rhythm alterations)
- antistamines (prolungation of the QT with ventricular hyperkinetic arrhythmias)
- sulphamides (allergic myocarditis)
- estro-progestins (increase of blood pressure)
- anti-secretory drugs eg., H_2 cardiac receptors blockess (hypokinetic arrhythmias)
- some anorectics eg. phenfluramina, dexphenfluramine (considered responsible for pulmonary hypertension)
- anabolic steroid (negatively condition the lipid profile and blood pressure)
- cocaine (responsible for coronary spasm and adrenergic sensitization)

References

1. Alpert MA, Lambert C., Boyd E. et al (1994) Effect of weight loss on ventricular mass in nonhypertensive morbidly obese patients. Am J Cardiol 73:918-921
2. Atanassov PG et al (1992)Pulmonary hypertension and dexfenfluramine. Lancet 339:436
3. Braunwald (1992) Heart disease. W.B. Saunders Company, Philadelfia
4. Brent GA (1994) The molecular basis of thyroid hormone action. N Engl J Med 331:847-853
5. Caldarone G, Giampetro M (1992) La prescrizione dell'attività fisica nelle malattie dismetaboliche. Serie Documenta Geigy in Medicina dello Sport, Ciba Geigy
6. Cecil (1992) Textbook of Medicine. W.B. Sunders Company, Philadelfia
7. Harrison's Principles of Internal Medicine. Mc Graw-Hill, Inc., New York, 1992
8. Huges DG et al (1989) Cardiovascular effects of H2-receptor antagonists. J Clin Pharmacol 29:472
9. Kennedy M (1990) Athletes, drugs and adverse drug reactions. Adv Drug Reaction Bull 143:536

10. Lange LA et al (1989) Cocaine-induced coronary artery vasoconstriction. N Engl J Med 321:1557
11. Schlant RC (1987) Electrophysiologic studies and unexplained palpitations. Circulation 75 (Suppl 3):159-160

IOC Banned Drugs and their Effects on the Cardiovascular System

C. Montemartini, G. Iraghi

Divisione di Cardiologia, IRCCS Policlinico S.Matteo, Pavia, Italy

Drugs Used for Doping Affecting the Cardiovascular System

Doping is defined as the administration or intentional use of substances external to the body, however they are introduced, or as measures taken by an athlete before or during a sporting event with the aim of artificially and illegally improving his sporting performance [18]. Physical performance is physiologically activated by means of the intense stimulation of all or nearly all the organs or apparatuses of the human body. This is particularly true for the cardiocirculatory system. There is no activity which does not require the immediate support of blood circulation, and so any substance capable of ergotropically modifying the physical performance has to act by stimulating the cardiocirculatory system. Many of them are normal deposit-releasing chemical mediators of cardiovascular ergotropic stimuli, that are usually synthesised and metabolised in the human body, but the majority are substances which are not present physiologically but can indirectly stimulate active cardiac and vessel receptors. In the first group, the stimuli are physiologically similar to those which normally occur during training sessions designed to improve gradually the responses of neuromodellers and so their artificial introduction into the circulation differs from normal physiology only in terms of their sudden effect and the lack of preparation on the part of the body as a whole; the substances in the second group have a reflex action which is accompanied by the large number of side effects which are themselves toxic for the organism.

In 1993, the International Olympic Committee's Medical Commission drew up a long list of substances which includes all clinical formulas whose use, alone or in association with others, can be considered as doping. These substances can be broadly classified into more or less homogeneous groups that have different effects on the cardiovascular apparatus, but, given that these stimuli are not physiological, they can all cause harmful side effects which may have immediate or later negative influence on an athlete's health.

Doping Classes

A. Stimulants	C. Anabolic agents	E. Peptide hormones
B. Narcotics	D. Diuretics	and analogues

Doping Methods

A. Blood doping (as far as the category of doping methods is concerned, it can said that only the method of blood transfusion could have some marginal effect on the circulation).

B. Pharmacologiocal, chemical and physical manipulation (the manipulations of the champion do not concern the present article).

Drug Classes Subject to Certain Restriction

A. Alcohol
B. Marijuana
C. Local Anesthetics
D. Corticosteroids
E. Beta -blockers.

Stimulants Releasing Noradrenaline from the Depot Vesicles of the Adrenergic Nerves (Presynaptic Nerve Endings).
They include substances with various clinical formulas, but they all have an intensive stimulating effect on the sympathetic nervous system (Table 1).

1) Indirect sympathomimetic agents act by releasing noradrenaline into the circulation. They provoke intensive sympathetic stimulation.

2) Tryciclic antidepressant, non-selective monoamine oxydase (MAO) inhibitors.

3) Centrally acting respiratory analeptics that stimulate the sympathetic nervous by reflex action.

Table 1. A- Stimulants

amfepramone	cocaine	furfenorex	phendimetrazine
amfetaminil	cropropamide	mefenorex	phenmetrazine
amineptine	(component of Micoren)	mesocarbe	phentermine
amiphenazole	dimetamfetamine	methamphetamine	phenylpropanolamine
amphetamine	ephedrine	methoxiphenamine	pipradol
benzaphetamine	etaphedrine	methylephedrine	prolintane
caffeine	ethamivan	methylphenidate	propylhexedrine
cathine	etilamfetamine	morazone	pyrovalerone
chlorphentermine	fencamfamin	nlkethamide	strychnine
clorbensorez	fenetylline	pemollne	
clorprenaline	fenproporex	pentetrazol	

4) Analeptics and cardiokinetic agents, smooth muscle relaxants (caffeine) directly stimulates the cortical part of the brain and increases exercise tolerance and psychological performance. The circulatory effects of caffeine are: tachycardia, premature ventricular beats, dilation of arterioles, vasoconstriction of the cerebral vascular bed.

5) Direct sympathomimetic agents: beta-agonists, alpha/beta agonist (clorprenaline). The stimulation of beta adrenergic receptors leads to calcium channels opening with increased inotropic effect and decreased dromotropic and chronotropic effect. The stimulation of alpha receptors leads to vasoconstriction, tachycardia and increased inotropic effect.

6) Synthetic centrally acting respiratory analeptics which have a similar action to those in group 3.

7) Non steroidal anti-infiammatory drugs (NSAIDs), which have a reflex stimulating action on the sympathetic system especially when used at high doses. They are not used for doping but they can give rise to positive results when tested in organic samples.

8) Central stimulants which have the same action as the substance.

9) Centrally stimulating alkaloids (strychnine) which increase the reflex excitability of the central nervous system. They improve reflexes/muscular tone, strength, stimulate breath, increase arterial pressure.

The way these substances affect the cardiovascular system depends on their stimulation of alpha or beta1-receptors. Alpha and beta1-receptors are mainly responsible for cardiovascular activity, whereas beta2-receptors mainly affect the respiratory system. The effects of stimulants on the cardiovascular system are due to the release of noradrenaline (Table 2). The literature describes cases of sudden death, major infarction and arrhythmic accidents due to the abuse of stimulants of sympathetic system [2, 19].

Table 2. Cardiovascular effects of noradrenaline

1.	Activation of cardiac beta receptors
2.	Activation of vascular alfa receptors
3.	Increase or decrease of cardiac output
4.	Increase of total pheripheral vascular resistence
5.	Increase of left ventricular after load
6.	Increase of the cerebral and coronary blood flow
7.	Decrease of blood flow in all the other districts
8.	Increase of myocardial oxigen consumption
9.	Possible arrythmogenic effect
10.	The effects on sino-atrial node may be maschered by reflex vagal bradicardia

Analgesics And Narcotics (Table 3)

Table 3. Analgesics and narcotics

alfaprodine	diidrocodeine	nalbufine
aniledrine	dipipanone	penthazocine
buprenorfine	etoeptazine	petidine
codeine	ethylmorphine	phenazocine
destromoramide	levorfanolo	trimepiridine
destropropossiphene	methadone	
diamorfine (heroin)	morphine	

These are substances with a morphine-like action that are not used for their stimulating action, but for their principal pharmacological activity of relieving pain. However, their multiple side effects may also represent an ergotropic stimulant by removing the impotence or functional limitations related to the presence of pain. The cardiovascular action of morphine and similar drugs is sustained by the inhibiting effect it has on the release of acetylcholine from both pre-and post ganglion fibres, which therefore hampers the propagation of parasympathetic stimuli. It is their euphoric effect that can be taking advantage of in the case of doping, but this is counterbalanced by their depressant effect on the respiratory centres, which are rendered much less sensitive to changes in CO_2 and are therefore no longer capable of modifying the hypercapnea caused by muscular effort. At therapeutic doses, they have hardly any effect on the circulation; but at high doses, they can lead to tachicardia and hypertension and, at the highest doses, to bradicardia and hypotension due to the depression of the superior centres.

Table 4. Steroids and anabolic agents

bolasterone	methyltestosterone
boldenone	nandrolone
clostebol	norethandrolone
dehydrochlormethyltestosterone	oxandrolone
fluoxymesterone	axymesterone
mesterolone	oxymetholone
metandienone	stanozol
metenolone	testosterone

Steroids And Anabolic Agent (Table 4)
1) Androstane derivatives with marked anabolic activity.
2) Estrone derivatives without a very pronunced androgenous effect.
3) Androgens which enhance muscle trophism and have androgenous effects.

At high doses, these have a vasodilating effect and all of them cause water retention. They increase CK-B levels but without ECG changes or cardiovascular symptoms [12]. They can be considered harmless if their use is not continous [9], but cases of myocardial infarction and dilatative myocardiopathy in athletes chronically administered with anabolic agents have been reported [19], and the concomitant use of cocaine increases the possibility of cardiovascular risks. There are reports from Australia of two athletes receiving anabolic agents who died during training (one of hypertrophic heart disease, the other of myocarditis), and two other cases of non-fatal infarction in 1988 and 1990 [11]. Use and effects of these substances are very uncertain [4]. No difference in the size or function of the left ventricle was found when athletes taking anabolic agents were compared with controls [16]. Increases in coronary risk factors of hypertension and dyslipidemia have been documented [5], and thrombosis has also been described [7]. Bruno has described anatomic and functional changes, concluding that with regard to the cardiovascular system there are sure effects (hypercholesterolemia, water retention), probable effects (aggresiveness and reduction of the fatigue thresold), possible effects (arteriosclerosis), uncertain effects (myocardial infarction and stroke) and there has been one case of sudden death [13]. As it can be seen, the cardiovascular alterations due to the use of anabolic agents are not specific and opinions are also discordant.

Diuretics (Table 5)
On the basis of their mechanism of action, these can be divided into:
1) Carbonic anhydrase inhibitors, which depress the proximal reabsorption of sodium bicarbonate and therefore water discharge through sodium discharge.
2) Potassium sparers, which antagonise the action of aldosterone by favouring the elimination of sodium and the recovery of potassium.
3) Thiazides, which inhibit reabsorption in the ascending ansa and the first part of the distal tubules.
4) Ansa diuretics, which inhibit sodium reabsorption in the ascending branch of the ansa Henle.
5) Antialdosterone agents, which have the same effect as the substances in group 2).
6) Mercurials, which inhibit the rebsorption of sodium, chloride, potassium and water.
7) Sulphonamides, which have same action as the drugs in group 3).

The cardiovascular action of diuretics is represented by a reduction in mass due to the loss of water and subsequent inspissatio sanguinis. The first group also cause acidosis and hyponatremia, with mild hypotension, hypokalemia and pronounced arrhytmias. At ECG, the P wave is high, there is a lengthened QTc interval, depressed T wave, low-voltage QRS, a lengthened P-Q interval and a

reduction of arterial pressure.
Groups 2) and 5) have a minimal diuretic action and may cause hyperkalemia.
Group 3) and 7) cause marked hypokalemia.
Group 4) causes hipokalemia and hemoconcentration.
Group 6), now obsolete and only for parenteral use, causes alkalosis and severe arrhythmias.

Diuretics can be used in sport to reduce body weight to allow athletes to fall within the weight limits of those sports which have them, or to dilute and rapidly eliminate the doping substances in such a way that they cannot be found in test samples.

Table 5. Diuretics

acetazolamide	diclofenamide
amiloride	ethacrinic acid
bendroflumethiazide	furosemide
benzothiazide	hydrochlorotiazide
bumetanide	mersalyl
canrenone	spironolactone
chlormerodrin	triamterene
chlortalidone	

Hormones

1) corionic gonadotropin, whose administration causes effects that are similar to those of the administration of testosterone

2) Adrenocorticotropic hormone (ACTH), which is equivalent to the administration of corticosteroids.

3) Somatotropic growth hormone, which is very inefficient, leads to many side effects (allergic reactions, diabetogenic effects, acromegaly) and is little used because of its high cost.

4) Erytropoietin, which regulates erythrocite synthesis. It can have the same effects as transfusions: that is, icrease blood mass and lead to hemoconcentration and polyglobulia, with their related effects on the circulation.

Doping Methods

A. Blood doping
B. Pharmacological, chemical and physical manipulation

Drug Classes Subject to Certain Restriction Includes Drugs or Substances that are Considered to have a Doping Effect Only at High Concentrations

A) Alcohol does not have major effects on the cardiovascular system (contrary to what normally believed). The most important effects of alcohol are on the metabolism and they only have secondary effects on circulation. Alcohol leads to increased levels of lactic acid, therefore determines acidosis interfering with the Krebs cycle and on the metabolism of the sympathetic amines. The final metabolite has a competitive action on the central nervous system transmission. Low doses of alcohol may reduce anxiety and therefore have a stimulating effect. It has a diuretic effect: the mechanism of action is a competition with the aldosterone system. It is considered a drug for doping only for the long lasting toxic effect.

B) Marihuana is not forbidden and has very little cardiovascular effects.

C) Local anaesthetic drugs. If used at high dose, they may have the same effects as analgesics.

D) More or less the same concept applies to corticosteroids which can have the same effect as anabolic agents:

E) Beta blockers may have very peculiar effect on the cardiovascular system since they have a depressing effect. They are not used as doping drugs except for particular sports. Indeed if used for therapeutic reasons it may be contraindicated to practise some sports.

Nowadays in the current clinical practice beta blockers are used be blocking selectively the beta1 receptor. These agents could be used in athletes for therapeutic reasons, especially for the prevention of premature ventricular beats. They may be used as doping in athletes to lengthem diastolic time (in shooters) and to limit possible negative effects due to anxiety and aggressiveness.

References

1. Antonaccio MJ (1980) Farmacologia clinica cardiovascolare. Martinucci Ed
2. Appleby M, Eischer M, Martin M (1994) Myocardial infarction, hyperkalemia and ventricular tachicardia in young male body builder. J Cardiol 44:171-174
3. Bruno M (1990) Gli steroidi anabolizzanti ed il loro abuso nella pratica sportiva Clin Ter 135:159-72
4. Celotti F, Negri-Cesi P (1992) Anabolic steroids. J Steroid Biochem Mol Biol 43:469-77
5. Cheever K, House Ma (1992) Cardiovascular implication of anabolic steroid abuse. J Cardiovasc Nurs 6:19-30
6. Di Biase G, Labriola E (1966) Le catecolamine e l'apparato cardiovascolare. Patrou Ed
7. Ferenchick GS (1991) Anabolic/androgenic steroid abusewith cardiomyopaty in atlet. Am J Med 92:562
8. Ferenchick GS (1991) Anabolic/andogenic steroid abuse and thrombosis, is there a connection? Med Hypotheses 35:27
9. Haupt HA (1993) Anabolic steroid and growth hormone. Am J Sport Med 21:468-74
10. Katz AM (1981) Fisiologia del cuore. Cortina Ed
11. Kennedy MC, Lawrence C (1993) Anabolic steroid abuse and cardiac death. Med J Aust 158:346-8
12. Jensen LK (1994) BivizKninger oy dopingcontrol Ved lrug of anabolic steroid.

Vgeskr-Laeger 156:58723-3

13. Luke JL et al (1990) Sudden cardiac death during exercise in a weight-ligter using anabolic steroids. J Forensic Sci 35:1441-7
14. Schimd P (1990) Der Einsatz von Beta-Rezeptors-Blockern in Leistungssport. Wien Med Wochenschr 140:184-8
15. Smith DA, Perry PJ (1992) The efficacy of ergonogenic agents in athletic competition. Ann Pharmacother 26:520-8
16. Thomson PD et al (1992) Left ventricular function is not impaired in weight-lifters who use anabolic steroids. J Am Coll Cardiol 9:278-82
17. Venerando A, Zeppilli P (1982) Cardiologia dello sport. Masson Ed
18. Vecchiet L, Calligaris A, Montanari G, Resina A (1990) Trattato di medicina dello sport applicata al calcio. Menarini Ed
19. Welder AA, Melchert RE (1993) Cardiotoxiceffects of cocaine and anabolic-androgenic steroids in the athlete. J Pharmacol-Toxical Methods 29:61-8
20. Zeppilli. Cuore d'atleta. Master Pharma Ed
21. Zinzen E, Clariys JP, Vanderstappen D, Vandenberg YJ (1994) The influence of triazolam and flunitruzepam an isokinetic and isometri muscle performance Ergonomics 37:69-77

Legal Implications of the Cardiovascular Evaluation of Athletes

M. Di Luca

Department of Medical Law, University "La Sapienza", Rome, Italy

In 1950 a special health protection law was introduced into the Italian legal system. According to this law professional and amateur athletes, who are regularly paid or practise sporting activities generally regarded as severe and dangerous, are obliged to undergo medical eligibility checks as a necessary qualification to practise sports. This law is the result of the application of art. 32 of the Constitutional Law of the Italian Republic approved in 1948.

The meaning of the constitutional provision is very clear: the health of the individual citizen and of the whole community is a form of public interest and the State must ensure citizens' health protection in all contexts of life, including work and sports activities.

On the track of the constitutional provision, another law was issued, still in force today, the 26 october 1971 Law, n° 1099, concerning Healt Protection of Sporting Activities. This law extends the requirement of selected medical checks and periodical fitness check-up to "any one who intends to practice or already practices athletic sporting activities". The health protection system, as regards the sporting community, has been improved through a number of Decrees issued by the Health Department.

This protection system singles out four groups of the sporting population: agonistic, non agonistic, professional and handicapped athletes. The classification based on the different health risks of the sporting activity which is determined by the heaviness of the activity itself.

Anyway, all athletes and people wanting to practise sports are obliged to undergo preventive and periodic check ups in order to obtain a certificate of eligibility attesting that the patient can practise sports without running health risks and that he or she does not suffer from pathological affections which can result in illness or death.

During the diagnosis and evaluation particular attention has to be devoted to cardiovascular diseases as they are the most frequent cause of athlete's death (sudden or non-sudden death).

The Health Department Decrees concerning sporting eligibility, both agonistic and professional, underline the fact that special attention has to be devoted to the evaluation of the cardiovascular system; for some sporting activities the certificate of eligibility requires a resting electrocardiographic exam and, sometimes, also a at stress ECG.

The most recent provisions regarding professional athletes' sporting eligibility have made obligatory an elettrocardiographic exam both at rest and at stress and a Doppler-ecocardiography.

The above mentioned provisions introduce many precise obligations for the sports physician who has to evaluate a patient's physical condition. Their omission determines, in juridicial terms, the nullity of the eligibility status given to the athlete.It should be noted that the Italian juridical system as relat to the above mentioned art. 32 of the Italian Constitution establishes the limit for anyone to dispose of his own life and physical integrity.

Art. 5 of the Civil Code forbids any activity which may permanently affect a person's physical integrity, while articles 579 and 580 of the Penal Code punish the murder of the consentient and the instigation of or help in committing suicide.

Besides this general limitation, there are also some areas of activity (work, school, sport, etc) in which the health-care of the individual and of the community is concretely protected by the Government through a program of preventive psycho-physical check-ups to which anyboby wishing to practise such activities is subjected.

After the check-up, the athlete can be allowed to or forbidden from performing such activities.

The issuing of the certificate of sport eligibility is the final and most important step of the Government health preventive program. Consequently, the athlete can practise sports activities in the context of official sport only if he is certified eligible by the sports physician. If the sports doctor does not issue the certificate of eligibility, then the athlete cannot start or continue practising sporting activities of any kind. The compulsory nature of the certificate as authorization to start sporting activities automatically involves the physician in juridical responsibility should either of the following events occur:

1) diagnosis or evaluation error by the sports physician during the medical examinations necessary to issue the certificate of eligibility;

2) damage (personal injury or death) of the athlete as a consequence of the physician's error.

As regards the first event (diagnosis or evaluation error), it should be clarified that the physician's error is juridically relevant only when it is done with malice aforethought; that is caused by unskillfulness, imprudence, negligence, or by non observance of coded rules of behaviour, as established in art. 43 of the Penal Code.

The sports physician might run into a malice aforethought error either when he carries out the medical examination or in the diagnostic or evaluation of the examination results.

An error made during the check up might hide clinical elements needed for a correct diagnosis of a disease of the cardiovascular system or relative to another organ, and which would compromise the issuing of the certificate.

Anyway, even if all proper medical examinations are carried out, the physician can still give wrong interpretation of the obtained data (diagnostic error).

Moreover, in spite of the exactitude of the clinical procedures and of the subsequent diagnosis, the sports doctor might run into an evaluation error by not giving appropriate importance to the diagnosed disease and authorising the athlete to practise sporting activities.

As regards cardiovascular diseases, the physician's error can occur in any of the above mentioned phases.

As regards the first phase, it should be noted that the omission of further clinical and instrumental investigations, over and above those suggested by the Health Department Decrees, can determine a malice aforethought error.

In fact, the Ministerial Decrees concerning health protection in the field of sporting activities establish that the sports physician can prescribe further examinations, in addition to the routine check ups, if there is a clinical suspicion which requires them.

This provision means that the doctor is obliged to analyse in depth all clinically unclear situations that might suspect the existence of a disease able to rendes the athlete unfit to practise any sport.

It should be pointed out that a recent jurisprudential tendency considers the omission of medical tasks (diagnostic and/or healing) a crime of omission of dutie, when the doctor acts in the person.

Now it is necessary to explain a fundamental characteristic of an Italian Public Official or Responsible of Public Service. It cannot be denied that the sports physician, working in the National Health Service or in stuctures associated with it, is under all the effects of a person charged with a Public Service. So, it is evident that possible negligences in diagnostics can be used to formulate imputations for omission of duties.

As regards the second and third phases (diagnosis and evaluation of the clinical and clinical-instrumental data), cardiovascular pathology is the most insidious in terms of the consequences which may arise from a diagnostic or evaluation error; it is well known that cardiovascular diseases are the main cause of sudden death among the sporting population.

It has to be underlined that the usual diagnostic (cardiovascular) parameters are not completely adequate to determine if an athlete is eligible or not; this is due to the particular adaptations in the athlete resulting from the performance of the sport activity.

The need to determine different cardiovascular parameters for sport eligibility diagnosis and evaluation was considered by cardiologists at least ten years ago, when they drew up a number of guide-lines, similar to the American (Bethesda Conference) and the Italian ones (Cardiological protocols for the judgement of sporting agonistic fitness).

What juridicial value can be given to such documents and, above all, how should the sports doctor behave regarding the indications contained in these documents?

Firstly, it is necessary to say that the main aim of these documents has been to provide practical indications to the sports doctor in an extremely difficult and complex subject, on the basis of the most up-to-date scientific acquirements.

The juridicial value of these documents can be understood from this fore-word: talking about indications coming from authoritative scientific assemblies.

Their aims are to lead the sports doctor to correct diagnostic-evaluation conclusions which are assimilable to dutiful codes of behaviour.

So, generally speaking, following such indications in diagnostic-evaluation base, the sports doctor can trust on a presupposition of correctness of his own acts juridically efficacious, so that he can be safe from prosecutings for responsability.

On the contrary, just because these indications dictated by the cardiological protocol come from scientifically authoritative sources, and because they are based on parameters of prudence and caution, it is advisable for the sporting doctor to step aside practically, because in the hypothesis of a damage it would be automatically a presumption of error committed by him since he has negletted a precise indication of the guide-line.

There is the need to clarify that in the scientific subject presumptions have often no bases, because in the area of sports cardiology, situations of very hard interpretation or not sufficiently known spread up, and in these cases the guide-lines can not give satisfactory indications.

The cardiologic protocols can be totally or partly dismissed by the sports doctor when a reasonable certainty exists, supported by uniquivocal and authoritative specialistic interpretations, that the clinical situation of the athlete does not expose him to risks in connection with the sporting exercise.

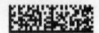